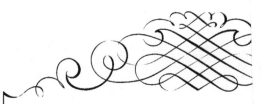
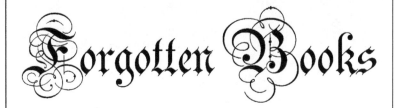

ISBN 978-0-260-23951-8
PIBN 11012683

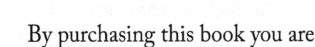

English
Français
Deutsche
Italiano
Español
Português

www.forgottenbooks.com

Mythology Photography **Fiction**
Fishing Christianity **Art** Cooking
Essays Buddhism Freemasonry
Medicine **Biology** Music **Ancient
Egypt** Evolution Carpentry Physics
Dance Geology **Mathematics** Fitness
Shakespeare **Folklore** Yoga Marketing
Confidence Immortality Biographies
Poetry **Psychology** Witchcraft
Electronics Chemistry History **Law**
Accounting **Philosophy** Anthropology
Alchemy Drama Quantum Mechanics
Atheism Sexual Health **Ancient History**
Entrepreneurship Languages Sport
Paleontology Needlework Islam
Metaphysics Investment Archaeology
Parenting Statistics Criminology
Motivational

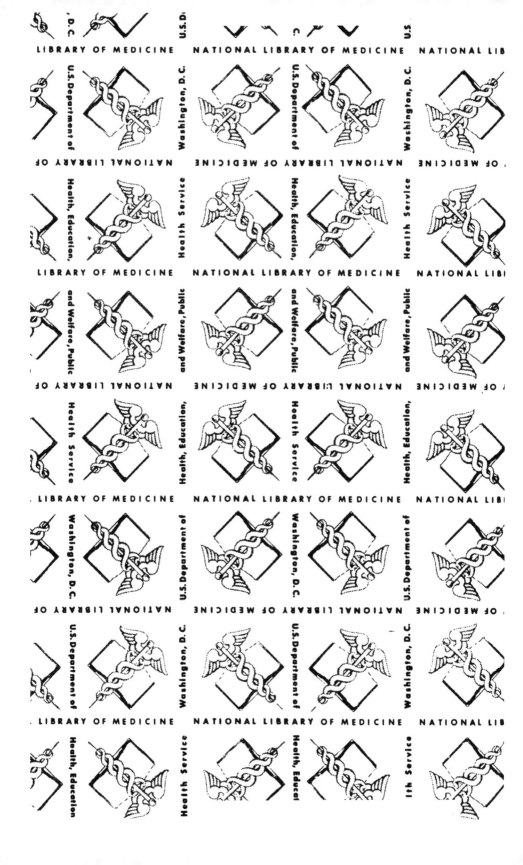

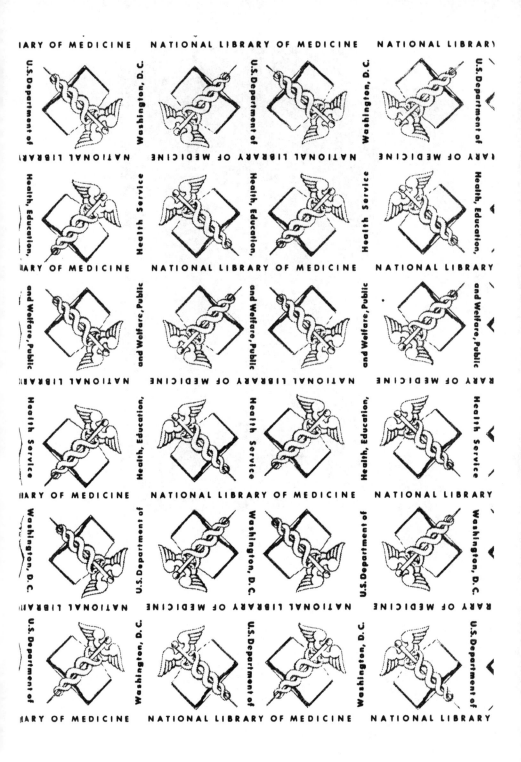

THE

POOR MAN'S FRIEND,

CONTAINING THE INFALLIBLE CURE

FOR THE BLACK TONGUE,

WITH ITS

CAUSES AND SYMPTOMS:

ALSO,

THE ONLY REMEDY KNOWN TO PREVENT THE
CONTAGION FROM ATTACKING THOSE IN
CHARGE OF THE PATIENT; WITH
THE TREATMENT FOR

MEASLES AND SCARLET FEVER,

AND

A COLLECTION OF

FIFTY VALUABLE REMEDIES

FOR VARIOUS DISEASES.

COMPILED FROM THE GERMAN BY
W. E. RICHTER, M. D.
BEDFORD COUNTY, PENNSYLVANIA.

PRINTED AT THE "NEWS OFFICE," HAGERSTOWN, MD.

1847.

PREFACE.

Actuated by motives of philanthropy, and fully convinced, also, that any thing which is beneficial to mankind at large ought to be fully and extensively known, and at the request of some of my respected friends of my vicinity, I have come to the conclusion of compiling the following pages; and as I commit them to the perusal and judgment of the community at large, I hope that any deficiency which may appear in the style may be balanced by the good intention of the author, in endeavoring to be useful to his fellow men, so far as in his power lies.

This collection of remedies and receipts contains some of the best preparations which have been used in Germany by celebrated physicians, and which have been kept secret for many years.

This work is not written in a scientific manner, because it never was intended for the professors of medical science, but for the community at large.—Therefore, in order to render it comprehensible to the unlearned, it is written in as plain a manner as possible. Should a learned critic cast his eyes over these pages, he is asked to spare them for the sake of those far distant from medical aid, and also for the sake of others unable to meet the exorbitant demands of physicians, who regard neither the voice of conscience nor the silent sufferings of the poor, but are ruled only by self-interest. Let him, therefore, as a

man of conscience, at least acknowledge the good intention of the author, instead of villifying every thing
that does not exactly agree with his judgment. Thus
I commit this little work to the public at large, hoping
that with the blessing of the Lord it may be the means
of saving the lives of many afflicted with that terrible
and dangerous disease called the "Black Tongue; and
if it should only be the means of saving one patient
from a sudden death and unprepared appearance before
the Almighty's Bar, the author will think himself rich-
ly repaid for his labor; for at best, the words of the
Apostle, " What is your life ?—it is even as a vapor,
that appeareth for a while and then vanisheth away,"
are but too true.

A strict and scrupulous adherence to the treatment
prescribed for the cure of the " Black Tongue" (so
called) is absolutely necessary and required in order
to expect a favorable result. Then, and then only,
the cure prescribed, if taken in time, will prove itself
to be infallible, as it has been in the hands of the
author, which the surrounding community of his resi-
dence have been pleased to certify. Care is required
in procuring the exact medicines prescribed in the
different receipts, and if reasonable indications are followed by the application of proper remedies, and those
applications are guided by a sound and firm judgment,
then this little work will prove itself invaluable where
medical aid is not at hand, or too expensive to be procured: In this the intention and object of the author
will be accomplished, and some service will have been
rendered by him to his contemporaries.

THE AUTHOR.

RECOMMENDATIONS.

We the undersigned inhabitants of Bethel, and the surrounding Townships of Bedford County, Pennsylvania, do certify that a disease generally known by the name of the BLACK TONGUE has visited our neighborhood more or less, ever since the year 1843, and has proved fatal in every case, baffling the skill of our best Physicians. In the year 1844 Dr. W. E. Richter located himself in Warfordsburg, and has from that time to the present administered to all afflicted with that dreadful disease in our neighborhood, and has, with the blessing of God, been successful in every case, having attended in his extensive practice a great many, of which he has not to our knowledge lost a single patient. As he is about publishing his mode of treatment of this awful disease, we therefore recommend it as worthy of the attention and generous patronage of the citizens of every section of the United States, and we have in witness thereof set our hand writing hereunder, at Warfordsburg, Bethel Township, Bedford County, Pa., the 10th day of March, A. D. 1847.

Obadiah Graves,	Thomas Rutherford,
Elizabeth Mann,	Eleanor J Thomas,
George Fields,	Harriet Morgret,
Jared Hanks,	Benjamine Gale,
Jason Hanks,	Benjamine Charlton,
Samuel Carnell,	David Rowland, Esq.
Joseph Bernhard,	George Morgret,
Ephraim Garland,	Thomas Robinson,

Benjamin Mellott,
John Stillwell,
Job Morgret,
Dennis Dannels,
John Dannels,
Abner Rowland,
Joseph Bernhard, Jr.
Rev. Jacob Watters,
Samuel Winter,
Joseph Mellott,
Paul Van Cleve,
Wm. W. Kirk,
Joseph Charlton,
John Rutherford,
James R Howell,
Francis Milliken,
Owen Rutherford,
James B. Orr,
John Bryner,
James Clark,
Elliot McCullock,
John Watt,
Moses Gregory,
Sarah Milliken,
Joseph Brewer,
Amos Dicken,
Robert McClelland,
Joseph Pittman,
Asberry Akers,
Jacob Fisher,
Moses Whitford,
George Smidt,
John Charlton,
James M. Powell,
Jacob Hull, Jr,
Dan Cook,
John E. Knable, Esq.
Henry Fite,
Lemuel Gorden,
James Hughes, Esq., Representative of Juniatta Co
Pa., in 1837 and 1838.
J. J. Kirk,
James C. Hughes,
Samuel Hooper,
Thomas M. Hedden,
Samuel Hedden,
Tobias Strasbaugh,
Gerald Moran,
William Mason.

This is to certify, that the men who have subscribe
their names to the foregoing publication, are men
good character and responsibility in our neighbo
hood. Witness our hands and seals, this 17th d
of March, A. D. 1847.

JOHN FISHER, J. P.   [L s.]

JACOB BERNHARD, J. P.   [L. s.]

Pennsylvania, Bedford County, ss :

I, JOSEPH B. NOBLE, Prothonotary of the Co

of Common Pleas for said County, certify that John Fisher and Jacob Bernhard, Esquires, whose names are subscribed to the foregoing Certificate, were on the date thereof, and now are, acting Justices of the Peace in and for said County, (residing in the Township of Bethel,) duly commissioned and qualified so to act, and further I certify that the signatures purporting to be theirs are genuine.

In testimony whereof I have hereunto set my hand [**L. S.**] and affixed the Seal of said Court at Bedford the 23d day of March, A. D. 1847.

JOSEPH B. NOBLE, Prothonotor.

CERTIFICATES.

This is to certify, that in the year 1845, in the month of August, a boy who was living with me, about sixteen years old, was afflicted with the (at that time in our neighborhood prevailing) disease called the Black Tongue; during three days little hopes were entertained of his recovery, but by the Lord's blessing, under the care and treatment of Dr. W. E. Richter, he was restored to health again. And as Dr. Richter is about publishing the mode of his treatment, I can therefore, and will cheerfully, recommend it to the attention and patronage of the people of the United States. Given under my hand and seal, in Bethel Township, Bedford County, Pennsylvania, the 19th day of March, 1847.

JAMES M. POWELL. [l. s.]

This is to certify, that in the year 1846, two of my children were afflicted with the Black Tongue, and were attended by Dr. W. E. Richter, and with the Lord's blessing they both recovered. I therefore recommend his treatment to the public at large, as worthy of their attention. Given under my hand and seal, this 19th day of March, 1847, in Bedford Co., Pennsylvania. JOHN MORGRET. [l. s.]
DANIEL DANIELS, Witness.

This is to certify, that during the year 1846, three of my children, from the age of six years to the age of eighteen, two boys and one girl, was afflicted with a disease called, generally, the Black Tongue, and by the blessing of God, under the treatment of Dr. W. E. Richter they all recovered. And as he is about publishing his mode of treatment of this dangerous disease, I therefore cheerfully recommend it, because it has been the means of saving many lives in our vicinity, and deserves the attention and patronage of the people of the United States. Witness my hand and seal, in Belfast Township, Bedford County, Pa., the 11th of March, 1847.

JOB MORGRET. [L. S.]

This is to certify, that during the year 1816, one of my daughters, a young woman of about twenty-one years of age, was taken sick with a disease generally called the Black Tongue, but by the blessing of God, under the treatment of Dr. W. E. Richter, she recovered again; and as I hear he is about publishing the mode of his treatment, I therefore cheerfully recommend it to the attention and patronage of the people of the United States. Witness my hand and seal, in Bethel Township, Bedford County, Pa., the 19th of March, 1847.

JOHN FISHER, J. P. [L. S.]

This is to certify that in the year 1845, my family was afflicted with that appalling disease called the Black Tongue; being ignorant of the nature of this disease, and thinking it to be nothing more than a common sore throat, I thought it unnecessary to call in a physician for several days, but my child growing worse, I called in Dr. Wilson, of Hancock, the next day I called on Dr. W. E. Richter, but the disorder having gone too far, this child died. The rest of my family was yet well. A few days after, two other of my children were attacked, Dr. Richter was called on immediately, and by the blessing of God, under the treatment of Dr. W. E. Richter they both recovered. I believe that his mode of treatment of this disease is nearly infallible if taken in time, and his publication is worthy of the attention and patronage of all the people of the United States. Witness my hand and seal this 11th day of March, 1847, in Bethel Township, Bedford County, Pennsylvania.

WILLIAM BISHOP, [L. s.]

Representative of Bedford Co., Pa., during the sessions of the Legislature of the years of 1844 and '45.

This is to certify, that in the summer of 1846, two of my children were afflicted with a disease called the Black Tongue, which was at that time greatly prevailing in our neighborhood. I made immediate application to Dr. W. E. Richter, and with the Lord's blessing, under his treatment they both recovered. I think it but justice to say, that since he intends to publish the mode of his treatment, it deserves the attention of the public, and his publication ought to receive the patronage of the people of the United States. Given under my hand and seal, this 19th day of March, 1847, in Bethel Township, Bedford County, Pa.

JOSEPH MELLOTT. [L. s.]

This is to certify, that my wife was in 1846 afflicted with the so called Black Tongue. I employed Dr.

W. E. Richter, and under his treatment, by the blessing of God, she was restored to health again. I cheerfully therefore, since he has been so successful in our
County in curing this disease, recommend the publication of his treatment as worthy of the attention of
the people of the United States. Witness my hand
and seal, this 19th day of March, 1846.

NICHOLAS BLESINGER. [L. s.]

The most common cause which predisposes a person in such a manner that the contagion will take
hold on his system, is weakness, and all causes which
can or may bring on weakness or a debilitated state
of the whole system; as for instance, inclination to
cattarhs, scorbutic and scrofulous disposition, or tendency of all the fluids to the body; low, marshy situ-
ations, where the air is very often damp, where a great
many people live in the neighborhood of swamps; also
very dry and hot weather in the summer, causing the
stagnation of running water; uncleanliness, unwhole-
some nourishment taken in the stomach; long con-
tinned want of vegetable diet, a particular epidemical
constitution of the air, which may have been brought
on by a great heat following the overflowing of waters
or running streams, or it may be brought on after a
battle in time of war, when there has been a great
deal of blood shed of man and brute;—in that line, or
under that head, might also be brought the evapo-
rations of graveyards in crowded cities, or the evapo-
rations of slaughter houses, which may have a tendency to infect the air with a poison, injurious to the
system and health of mankind.

Dr. De Haen mentioned, in his writings, a large
well in Holland, which was no longer in use, into
which was thrown, during several years, all kinds of
offall and dirt of a town close by, and also from the
neighboring villages, with a view of shutting it up

gradually in this manner. All at once a contagious fever, of a putrifying nature, made its appearance in that neighborhood, proving very fatal to the inhabitants; after many trials for its cure, and many searches for its cause, it was at last found to be produced by the evaporation of this well. Hands were employed to shut up the great opening of this well, and soon after the fearful epidemic ceased. Furthermore it is certain that epidemic diseases will spread more rapidly among the poorer class of the inhabitants of large cities, because they generally live in small houses, and narrow, dirty streets, than it will in the country where the air is more pure, and the people live more scattered and separate. From some of these causes a sharp poison is produced, which shows itself in an inexplicable manner, especially in the throat, or else in the windpipe, sometimes in both at once, and there by degrees establishes, especially if a predisposition to it exists in the system, that terrible disease, which is appalling in its symptoms and so dangerous and fatal in its consequences. The contagion spreads from family to family, from place to place, (which may be done in different ways and manners, either through clothing, or by sending goods from one town to another, which helped to spread the Cholera in some countries in Europe, during the years of 1831 and 1832,) till a complete epidemic is established, or it may be spread in innumerable different ways and manners. Be this as it may, it is beyond doubt that this sickness is contagious, in proportion as an individual is more or less predisposed to its influence.

This disease does not only affect certain constitutions, nor at a certain age only; neither does it appear at certain seasons; but children, the female sex, and weakly persons, are more apt to be afflicted with it than the male sex and robust persons; although, it is granted, there have been exceptions, when robust persons have also been afflicted and carried off suddenly with this disease; and it has been observed to be more prevalent in the fall and the commencement of winter, than in the spring and summer. There has happened cases of it during all seasons of the year, even in the midst of winter, when there was snow on the ground to the depth of eighteen inches. It is not thought necessary to trace this matter any further, and I shall therefore proceed to give a description of the symptoms of the disease.

SYMPTOMS.

The throat in most cases suddenly becomes of a shining red color, appearing as if there was much inflamation, accompanied with slight pain and a feeling of burning disagreeable sensation, along with more or less stiffness of the neck, which symptoms often deceive through their mildness, until the patient is past all recovery.

Upon these red inflamed-looking places there soon appear, here and there, irregular white, ashy-colored spots, which are often surrounded with a redish looking ring. These spots get larger and greater in size, run together and suddenly they are changed into white, blue, or blackish looking scabs, of a gangrenous tendency, under which are hidden deep and broad ulcers, which will appear by close observation. From underneath these scabs, which cover these ulcers, there oozes out continually an acrimonious, bad smell-

ing fluid, which affects the neighboring parts and produces a stinking and highly contagious breath, which
will hardly ever be observed till these ulcers are formed, when the cadaverous smell of the breath will be
observable.

Sometimes it happens that there are small pimples
visible, of the appearance of blisters, filled with a yellow or greenish-looking fluid, which, however, quick-
ly are changed into ulcers and spread themselves
deeper in the throat, and also upwards to the nose.
Out of the nose and mouth commences to run a highly offensive, yellowish or greenish matter, of a very
corroding nature, and sometimes even blood. The
disease sometimes attacks the windpipe; and suddenly spreads downward to the lungs; all the parts which
lay above the stomach and the lungs are attacked, the
skin in the inside of the mouth and throat becomes
separated and falls off in putrid pieces, about which
time begin to appear, in the mouth and throat, dark
red and blackish-looking pieces of flesh, having an
appearance as if the flesh had been ripped with a saw.
The swelling of the surrounding external parts sometimes, reaches a great and fearful height at this period,
threatening suffocation ; from this cause it is, that although there was at first little difficulty in swallowing food, the patient can only now do it with difficulty, or not at all. The drawing of the breath is
also difficult, and power of speech begins to fail ; the
patient is hoarse, coughs, sneezes and speaks through
the nose with a deep hollow sound, and often complains of a sharp stinging pain in the throat, under the
breast bone. Sometimes a pain in the stomach is felt,

with an intolerable aversion to food, accompanied by
an uneasy sickness in the stomach, and sometimes
vomiting. If any of the corroding matter, which
oozes out of the ulcers in the throat, is swallowed,
which often happens, especially in children, it produces an agonizing pain in the stomach, accompanied,
perhaps, by a diarrhœa resembling flux, or bloody
stools mixed with matter, which corrodes the funda-
ment and its surrounding parts in the same manner
as the matter which runs out of the mouth and nose
corrodes the lips, cheeks, and hands of the patient,
and also the fingers and hands of the nurse. In some
cases it happens that there is running from the ear a
strong offensive-smelling matter, which may produce
deafness of one or both ears.

If the windpipe is affected, the patient in coughing
throws up pieces of the internal skin, mixed with
blood and a putrid slime. It is then that a shrill,
hoarse, or wheezing sound will be heard when the
patient draws his breath ; which sound is similar to
the sound that accompanies the drawing of the breath
of a patient afflicted with the croup.

The tongue is generally moist, appearing clean upon the extremity, but further back, towards the root,
it is covered with a yellowish or brownish-looking
coat, or it is covered with a thick whitish-looking
slime, or sometimes assumes the red appearance of
raw flesh.—The scabs in the throat sometimes fall
off, but are soon formed anew. Several parts may be
destroyed in this manner by these ulcers. If there is
any attempt made to swallow drink, it is rejected and
thrown out again through the nose. When mortifi.

eation is once finally and fully established, the pain
in the throat ceases, and the difficulty of swallowing
is in a manner removed, or at any rate, somewhat
lessened. Losses of blood may happen in different
ways at this period of the disease. In very desperate
cases there appears, sometimes, a swelling of the
whole neck, which may reach even down to the
breast, and, following this, a red-looking, much swollen face; at other times, a pale color of the face with
a mournful expression of countenance; red, watery
and sunken eyes; pressure and oppression, or a feeling of tightness around the regions of the heart; great
anxiety and restlessness; a weakness with inclination
to fainting ; a small, weak pulse ; pale, reddish, sometimes muddy-looking urine; sometimes a breaking out
of the skin, on the neck, breast, or arms, or on other
parts of the body; a giddiness of the head; a continued inclination to sleep; headache; delirium or raving;
a sensation of heaviness in the limbs ; a continued
sighing, with an expression of the countenance as if
there was great suffering; a stupified state of the mind,
in which the patient recognises no one ; and sometimes unusual liveliness, accompanied by much talk-
ing, or at least attempts to talk, which too often induce a vain hope of recovery. But death, in some
form, soon closes the scene. Sometimes, the patient,
with a few long-drawn sighs, breathes his last. At
others he is carried off in a raving delirium, or falls
quietly to sleep. Again, springing from his bed, in a
vain attempt to flee, he sinks and breathes his last.

If blood is drawn from a patient afflicted with this
disease, it looks generally very red, has no cousis-

tence at all, and is in a dissolved state. These appearances indicate a tendency to putrefaction, existing
in the fluids of the body, and the disease to be of a
very malignant nature.

Connected with all these symptoms is always more
or less fever, of an intermitting nature, which increases in violence towards night; this feverish state
either accompanies the beginning of the disease, or it
makes its appearance soon after the throat becomes
sore, and commences then with a shivering, trembling
and coldness of the extremities, and, perhaps, of the
whole body, which last but a short time, and then
are followed by a burning feverish heat of the whole
system, the skin remaining dry. Some times the fever
is, in the beginning, not so violent; but suddenly increases fearfully; at other times it commences vio-
lently, but soon looses its violence and apparently
ceases entirely. In the evening and at night the patient is generally worse; towards morning, after a
light sweat, he appears better. The fever accompanying this disease resembles in its nature and course
the nature of a malignant putrid fever. To be sure,
it may be changed in different ways and manners,
hrough different circumstances, causes and times, or
by the epidemical existence of the disease, and may
then assume different appearances. Sometimes it will
assume and produce symptoms nearly similar to those
of a bilious fever.

At times the disease may come on suddenly; at
other times by deceitful intermission, changing the
pulse but very little from a natural pulse; the thirst
is small; the pain in the throat inconsiderable; the dif-

ficulty of swallowing but little and trifling, as if no dangerous disease had taken hold of the patient. But be not deceived, lest your apparently safe situation prove your ruin. This disease is one of the most deceitful, and when the patient thinks himself most sure and safe, and fancies there is little danger, suddenly the symptoms change, and the disease assumes the terrible appearance above described, when all medical aid and human wisdom come too late. Therefore, persons should be very careful, and apply effectual means whenever any of the before mentioned symptoms make their appearance, for when once putridity of the mouth and throat sets in and drink is ejected through the nose, very little hope is left; while but a few hours before, medical aid could have accomplished a certain cure.

This disease is always dangerous, but may occasionally appear in a milder form, so that nature itself in a short time, in otherwise healthy persons, will effect a cure, but this is, indeed, a very rare occurrence. In most cases of a fatal issue, it proves fatal between the first and the fourth day; either in an apoplectic manner, or by a kind of fainting fit, or through inflamation of the brain, or excessive losses of blood from the lungs, nose or ears; or if in the female sex, from the parts of generation. Examination after death has shown the lungs covered with putrid, black, and blue looking spots, gangrenous ulcers in the bowels, and even torn entrails; but it may also, through its malignant consequences, prove fatal, after its main symptoms have disappeared; producing Dropsy, Consumption, Spitting of Blood, Diarrhoea, Suffocation and a host of other dangerous diseases.

Children, generally, are in greater and more sudden danger than adults. Death is often announced
by the appearance of dark, blue, black-looking spots,
which suddenly disappear again; also in the black
color of the internal parts of the mouth and throat;
swelling of the face, neck and the whole body; hic-
cups; fits; very pale, cadaverous face; voiding of very
clear, pale-looking urine; still delirium; sudden dis-
appearance of the matter which exudes from the nose
and mouth, or ears; excessive loss of blood; fainting;
cold extremity; involuntary stools; picking of the bed-
clothes, and in the air with the fingers, and a short
hurried, rattling breath. Sometimes death may take
place without any of these symptoms, or forerunning
signs, apparently only brought on by suffocation.

If the patient gets better, it takes place after mild
sweats have made their appearance, and a thick urine
is voided, which if left standing, will leave a sediment
in the bottom of the vessel. Also, a pealing-off of
the skin will be observed, more or less, upon the different parts of the body. The breathing becomes more
free; the fever and the heat decreases; the scabs in the
throat fall off; the matter in the throat assumes a mild
appearance and becomes less every day. The flesh
in the mouth and throat begins to look clean and natural; the ulcers disappear; the pulse is more regular;
the look of the eyes is enlivened, and the patient gains
in strength. Should there be a red-looking eruption
observed on different parts of the body, or all over it,
it may also be viewed as a favorable symptom, but
more common will be an itching in the skin, especially in adults, and the sickness in the stomach dis-

appears after the breaking of the skin. When the disease has existed epidemically, there has sometimes been observed the appearance of very disagreeable boils in the groins. One of the good signs, generally supposed to be so among European physicians, is said to be, when in the progress of the disease the neck gets very red externally, swells some and the skin commences to peal off. The duration of this disease is different in different subjects and different climates; it may last twelve or fourteen days and more, but often it is decided on the sixth or seventh day, for better or worse, if it does not sooner put an end to the patient's life.

However, this may differ in different epidemics; for individual and local causes, complications, and an epidemical constitution of the air, may sometimes make a great change and difference in the symptoms accompanying the beginning, progress and end of this disease; although much will always depend on the causes which produced it, the situation in which the throat is found, the nature of the fever accompanying it, and the influence which it may have upon the constitution of the patient, according as he is of a robust or delicate habit.

In the year 1778, there existed in Germany an epidemic of this disease which proved very fatal, especially to children afflicted with worms. This sickness, at that time, generally proved fatal on the sixth day, if the proper and necessary evacuations had been neglected. It was supposed to have been rendered more fatal by the influence which the worms and their slime exercised upon the fever through the progress of the disease.

We will now, without further reference to the history of this terrible disease, proceed to the exposition of the remedies proposed for its cure, which have never been known to fail if resorted to in season.

The first most necessary and pressing indication for the cure of this disease, points to vomiting, or remedies that will produce vomiting. The great use and benefit thereof has been proven by repeated experience. The violence and fatal progress of this disease has often been arrested by one single vomit; at other times it has given great ease to the patient, and has facilitated the subsequent cure. It is seldom that it will be necessary by other remedies to prepare the patient for the taking of a vomit, provided the help does not come altogether too late, and after the appearance of a powerful cramp in the parts affected; which certainly would have to be removed by external and internal mollifying medicines, under which head might come slimy drinks, sweetened with honey dissolved in vinegar, or the diluted juice of lemon, or small doses of Antimonial wine every half hour, till the cramp ceases; also, external applications may be used, such as warm poultices applied to the stomach, or fomentations of hot water or vinegar to the lower parts of it; also injections of sweet oil, or melted lard, and sweet milk. In all these preparations care must be taken not to bring on a diarrhœa. When the cramp has been removed, together with the great dryness, anxiety and pain, then a vomit will be given with the best and happiest result. But, as before stated, it will seldom be necessary to prepare a patient in that manner, as very seldom a cramp of that nature will be found which would forbid the administration of a vomit. Through a vomit

not only the unclean and foul stomach will be emp-
tied, but also the throat will be cleansed, the glands
enlivened, and the perspiration promoted; so that a
vomit will here answer four very desirable ends. (A
vomit for children up to fourteen years of age, may
consist of Antimonial wine, in doses according to
their age—above that age Ipecacuanha mixed with a
little tartar emetic may be given. See table and directions for administering it.) I have never in my
practice commenced the treatment of this disease in
any other manner than by giving an effectual vomit,
without regard to age or sex, and have always found
the best and most happy results to follow. Repeated
stools, without a vomit, cannot have the same good
effect produced by one effectual vomit—which, at any
rate, sometimes will perform one or two operations
downward. If there is no great indication contrary
to the administration of a vomit, and the disease has
not already gone so far that the patient's life only depends upon suddenly reviving the vital spirits, nothing else should detain us at any time during the progress of this disease, from administering an emetic,
and from repeating the same as often as necessary;
which may be known by much bitterness or nasty
taste in the mouth, like rotten eggs; or much weight
about the stomach, with a feeling of sickness or inclination to vomit; also, if the tongue has a brown
or yellowish looking coat, then the repetition of a
vomit would be of great benefit, and almost absolutely necessaay.

Besides the emetics, it is necessary that the patient
should have, daily, one or two passages by the stool,

which may be produced by giving him a small dose of calomel, followed by salts; (see prescription No. 3 & 4,) the dose to be governed by the age of the patient, as in the table and directions for the administering of physic.

Calomel will undoubtedly here have the preference over other kinds of physic; while, as in other fevers of a malignant putrid nature, it may happen that colliquative diarrhœas are brought on, proving hurtful if not fatal.

These diarrhœas, if they can be prevented at all, will be best guarded against by administering calomel, followed by mild opening remedies, such as salts, cream of tartar, or castor oil. Injections as before prescribed, may be given instead of calomel, once or twice a day; but I would prefer the calomel, having also the opinion of celebrated European physicians in its favor, such as Vogel, Hufeland, Grave, Tirsot and others.

It is certain that care is required in administering any medicines for the purpose of opening the bowels, always paying attention to the strength of the patient, the irritation of the bowels, (if such exists,) and the nature and foetid smell of the excrements voided, which generally have a highly offensive smell, similar to putrefaction. We must also remember that the weakness or debility of the patient, which may exist, may not have its cause or origin alone in the uncleanness contained in the bowels and stomach, but it is also to be sought in the tendency to putrefaction existing in the blood. However, from whatever cause this weakness may arise, it ought not to deceive us, nor deter us from the careful administration and repetition of mild opening remedies, so long as a hard swollen state of the stomach, together with a disagreeable rifting up of wind, pain in the bowels, headache, spells of delirium, passing cold sweats, disposition to sleep, and similar circumstances betray and point to the existence of bile, in a putrifying state, in the stomach and bowels; the removal of which is so much more necessary, as it promotes the tendency to putrefaction in the blood.

Under carefully guided and repeated evacuations of the stomach and bowels, the before mentioned symptoms, which may exist after one vomit and physic, will gradually disappear, and strength will be gained by degrees, especially if the patient drinks freely some acid beverage, made by mixing his drink with a little vinegar or sour wine, which will have a tendency to strengthen him.

After a vomit has been given the first and second time, a physic of a mild nature (see prescription No. 5 or 6,) preceded by a small dose of calomel, will answer all that can be expected. According as these medicines, which carry the bad matter and bile out of the body, have a greater or less effect, their dose must be either increased or decreased, which may be guided by considering the strength of the patient, the benefit derived from them at the time, and other circumstances.

The patient should use for his usual beverage, a drink of a sour, cooling and strengthening nature, such as weak lemonade; tea made of pounded or ground-barley; or blackberry juice mixed with vinegar and water; or a drink as prescribed in prescription No. 7, which drink ought to be given freely, though always remembering that the throat should be washed or gargled before swallowing any drink or food of any kind; for if that is neglected the ulcerated matter may be carried from the throat into the stomach. The diluted vitriolic acid, mentioned in prescription No. 7, is. one of the best remedies against putrefaction, second only, it may be said, to Peruvian bark, (Cortex Peruviana,) if taken in a sufficient quantity to produce an impression upon the system.

The calomel also, is a remedy deserving our greatest attention in this disease, for in the most desperate cases, when the best remedies failed, calomel and calomel alone was the means which saved the patient. It had to be given in repeated doses, sufficient to produce a slight salivation; the greater the existing tendency to putrefaction, the greater must be the doses of calomel.

Dr. Michaelis and Dr. Douglas both agree, that it has done wonders in the most hopeless cases, and Dr Bailey maintains the fact that none die upon whom salivation can be produced. Douglass also calls it a specific remedy for this disease, and in my own practice I have seen one very desperate case, in which calomel, given in sufficient quantity to produce a slight salivation, was the means of saving the patient's life when all else failed. Sec case No. 2.

What next deserve our attention are the neck and

throat; which must be closely attended from the beginning. Gargling is necessary, or if impracticable
from the debility or youth of the patient, injections
into the throat of cleansing remedies calculated to prevent or counteract putrefaction, may be used; or rags
dipped in some similar fluid may be used to wash the
mouth every three or four hours, and particularly before taking food or drink. The best remedies for
gargling or washing are, if the patient be a grown
person, a gargle made of gum myrrh and Cayenne
pepper; (see prescription No. 8,) or lime water; or
strong lukewarm vinegar; or red pepper tea sweetened with honey; and in younger persons, blackberry
juice with honey and vinegar, will answer the purpose. See prescription No: 9.

Often, however, in cases of small children no use
can be made of these gargles or remedies; as they are
difficult of management and can not be made sensible
of their danger. They will in consequence swallow
more or less of the putrid matter issued from the ulcers in the throat, which is undoubtedly the cause
why this disease is more fatal to children than adults.

The above mentioned strong gargles are only recommended if there are evidences of matter or ulcers
visible in the throat, which may be easily discovered
if the tongue is pressed down with the handle of a
spoon or a dull knife. As long as there are only redness and pain in the throat, with signs of inflammation, gargles of a different nature may be used, which
are less heating, irritating, or astringent than the a-
bove mentioned. The following will answer: tea of
sage, sweetened with honey; tea made of wheat bran;

flaxseed, blackberry juice, elder blossoms, or sweetened water; taking care, however, not to swallow any of it.

A direction suitable in all cases is not easy to describe; we ought, however, to be guided by the symptoms in the case, and as long as there are ulcers and matter visible, the gargles should be continued; for cleanliness of the parts is a great safeguard and absolutely necessary for safety. When the putrid nature of the ulcers is changed and better, the milder gargles may be used, in place of the stronger, sharper and more effectual.

To the same intent and purpose which the gargles answer inwardly, belong outward applications about the throat and neck; which may be made according to prescription No. 11. A mustard plaster may be applied under the chin around the throat, or a blister of Spanish flies may be laid on the back of the neck, and after having drawn there, it may be removed to the arm, half way from the elbow to the shoulder; and a blister drawn there, both of which must be well attended with poultices. (See directions for blistering.) Or the blister may be laid a second time, on the calves of the legs, until perfectly drawn. If the patient should complain of much burning pain unde the breast-bone, the blister may be applied there instead of upon the arms or legs. This has often given great relief and produced the most happy results.— The blisters have the tendency to draw from the throat and the surrounding parts the poisonous matter, or at least draw off some of the humours which feed the ulcers and sores in the mouth and throat.

Bleeding is seldom advisable in this disease, except it be in the very beginning, and then only if the patient is of a very plethoric habit, (full of blood.)— More commendable would be local blood evacuations, in the beginning of the disease, by cupping; though I never had recourse to either.

Should there be much hoarseness, and the patient complain of much heat in the throat, there may be given daily two or three doses of prescription No. 12, for a few days. But this will seldom be necessary if other directions are properly followed. I have only twice in many cases found it necessary, and then it was more with the intention of promoting perspiration, which was plainly indicated by a moist skin.

It is almost impossible to err in the application of the above mentioned remedies, if guided by reasonable indications and a sound judgment; which indications will be better comprehended by reading attentively the cases described hereafter. To make the matter more plain we will, after having thus extensively described the treatment of this disease, reduce it to five recapitulating heads, which, if judiciously persevered in, will effect a happy and speedy cure.

I. The first necessary remedy is a vomit. (See directions how to give it.) After the stomach is again settled, say about 12 or 16 hours after the vomit, give

II. A dose of calomel, regulated according to the age of the patient, and followed by a dose of salts, (if a grown person, a table-spoon-full will answer; if a child under 14 years old, one or two tea-spoons-full.) It may be necessary to repeat both vomit and physic in two or three days.

III. As soon as the throat is sore, gargling should be used every three or four hours; if ulcers and matter are visible, of the stronger gargles; if neither matter nor ulcers are visible, and there are only redness and pain, the gargles of the milder kind will answer. But always remember, that no food or drink is to be given at any time until the throat has been cleaned effectually by gargling or washing.

IV. One or more blisters will be necessary; first on the back of the neck or on the throat, and secondly, on the arm or calves of the legs. The blisters must be well attended. (See directions.) The liniment, No. 11, and the mustard plaster may be used before the blister is had recourse to; but I would always prefer an effectual remedy to an uncertain one; and therefore I would advise the blister at once.

V The drink of the patient may be as before mentioned. The diet should be of a light but nourishing nature. Cold water and rich food should be especially avoided. Also, fresh fish and eggs. I have seen patients recover in half the usual time, who used neither; while others who observed no abstinence paid dearly for their whistle, by greatly delaying their recovery.

Therefore, since experience has taught me, I have made it a practice to forbid, strictly, the use of cold water and strong diet, by patients afflicted with this disease. Other physicians may laugh at this, and they are perfectly welcome to do so, but they are not my masters. I speak conscientiously, guided by the experience of many years, and also. in accordance with the opinion of some of the best European physicians. Let others try the same, and if no benefit is derived from abstinence, then it is time enough to resort to ridicule. I am well aware of the fact that there are men among the vast number of physicians in our country, who will ridicule every thing that does not agree with their notions and judgment. But let it be remembered that their visions are obscured by ignorant prejudice. Let them, also, remember that the ideas held forth in these pages are sanctioned by other medical writers, of modern and ancient Europe—men of eminence and acknowledged science.

I shall now proceed to the description of a few of the great number of cases which came under my care and observation during the years 1845 and 1846; all of which were treated in the above described manner with one exception, that of a young lady, on accoun of an unforseen and unavoidable circumstance. But even that case, desperate and dangerously difficut, was, under the blessing of God, safely guided, and the lady restored to perfect health. (See case No. 2.)

CASE No. 1

A girl of about four years of age, attacked with the Black Tongue; throat very red and signs of ulcers; much anxiety and restlessness; fever more or less, through the day, always increasing towards evening and after night; loss of appetite; a coated brown looking tongue; swallowing difficult and sometimes painful; stiffness of the neck and inclination to vomit, together with headache; bowels in a costive state.

A vomit was immediately given, consisting of An-timonial wine, which brought up a quantity of greenish-looking matter or bile, and produced also one or two passages downward. This was in the morning. Gargles of the milder kind were used during the day, and in the evening a blister was put on the throat and a dose of Calomel given, which was followed the next morning by Salts. Three or four very offensive stools of a blackish color were effected. The blister had drawn well, it was poulticed attentively and the gargles were continued. Upon the next day, in the afternoon, the vomit was repeated, there being much appearance of matter in the throat with tolerable high fever. About twelve or sixteen hours after the vomit, another dose of Calomel was given, followed in about four hours by a second dose of Salts. The patient was directed to drink sour drinks, composed of vinegar, water and honey. The blister at this time was put on the back of the neck; the physic operated well, the stools having yet a putrid smell, and darkly colored. The breath was also bad..—During the night a tolerable quiet sleep ensued, together with a slight perspiration. After that time she commenced mending rapidly; the gargling of the throat and the poulticing of the blister was still continued; and in about three days more the physic was repeated, after which the throat gradually assumed a natural appearance; and in about eight days the patient was free from the disease and beyond danger.

CASE No. 2.

A young lady of about eighteen years old, of a spare habit and delicate constitution, taken with the

same disease; for several days used domestic remedies without effect. About the sixth day I was called on to see her, and found her in a pitiful situation.
A pale, mournful countenance; a small, weak pulse;
very bad, putrid-looking ulcers in the throat, having
scabs of a blackish color; a very offensive breath, perceptible as soon as the room was entered; a sick stomach, together with loss of appetite; great dejection
of the mind; costiveness of the bowels; restlessness
and disturbed sleep at night; weakness of the eyes,
so that she could not endure the light; some headache; more or less fever through the day; difficulty
in swallowing and stiffness of the neck. A vomit
was immediately given which brought away much
bilious-looking, offensive matter. A dose of Calomel
was next administered, the strongest gargles of Myrrh
and Cayenne pepper were ordered to be used, and a
blister was put on the back of the neck; the patient
being accustomed to smoking was allowed to smoke,
which she said gave her ease; about the third day after, the vomit and physic were repeated, and the patient ordered to drink acid drinks. The symptoms
appeared favorable, when unfortunately, as the time
of her catamenia arrived, she was suddenly attacked
with a violent flooding; which, in her already weak
condition, produced a great and fearfully dangerous
prostration. Four grains of Opium were mixed with
forty grains of Sugar of Lead; and divided into twelve
powders, one of which was directed to be taken every
half hour until the flooding ceased. After taking four
of the powders she was relieved of the flooding, but
excessive costiveness had been produced, which perhaps increased the already existing tendency to putre-

faction. The consequence was that her throat grew
worse; her breath became so offensive that persons
could scarcely remain in the room; pieces of putrid
flesh began to separate themselves from the inside of
the mouth, which appeared as if it had been lacerated
with a saw; spots of a putrid, blackish color appeared in all parts of the mouth; there was great weakness;
a hardly perceptible pulse; headache, danger of fainting. Under these circumstances the strongest kinds of
gargles were used as often as possible, and doses of
Calomel repeated hourly, which soon produced a
slight salivation, upon the appearance of which the
patient immediately began to mend, her throat gradually getting better. By continued gargling and attention to the regular evacuation of the bowels, she
finally recovered. No cold water was allowed during the progress of her sickness.

CASE No. 3.

A boy of about twelve years of age was taken sick
during the summer of 1846; had been sick about four
days when I saw him for the first time. I found his
throat somewhat swollen, and having small white
spots on both sides; a sick stomach, with considerable headache; high fever, but dry skin; anxiety and
restlessness; loss of appetite; difficulty in swallowing,
with some stiffness of the neck; his tongue was coated with a yellowish brown coat; his pulse 110; his
eyes inflamed.

A vomit was given of Antimonial wine, followed by
a dose of Calomel and Salts; a blister was put on the
back of the neck, and red pepper mixed with vinegar
and honey, used as a gargle. In forty-eight hours the

vomit and physic were repeated; after that he appeared to be getting better; his throat did not look as bad as before; his pulse was better; his headache was gone. He was ordered to continue the gargling and take more Salts the next morning. That night, the window having been accidentally left open, he caught cold, and in the morning was much worse. His throat at noon appeared full of matter; fever had increased; sickness in the stomach prevailed; inclination to sleep; also difficulty of breathing; running of matter from the nose; bowels costive, having neglected to take the Salts as directed; and breath offensive. A dose of Calomel was given, followed by Salts; the blister laid on the calves of the leg; the gargles continued, and sour wine, in a diluted state, was ordered to be given. In three days the physic was again repeated; after which his throat gradually assumed a natural appearance, his fever altogether disappeared and he recovered. The blister on the leg, however, remained unhealed about four weeks longer; having been suffered to remain on too long.

CASE No. 4.

The sister of the above mentioned boy, about ten years of age, took sick about the same time. She had very high fever, which caused delirium; a loathing of all kind of food; complaint of weight about the stomach; tongue coated with a white-looking slime; difficulty in swallowing, and the appearance of small white-looking ulcers in the throat; much headache; inflamed eyes and restlessness.

A vomit was given, followed by a good dose of Calomel; a blister put on the back of the neck, the mild gargles directed to be used, and in forty-eight hours the vomit and physic repeated. Two days after, a dose of Salts was given, after which her throat began to assume a natural appearance, and all the symptoms of the disease disappeared; she having fallen into a light perspiration after the operation of the second physic. In six days she was again well.

CASE No. 5.

A lady of about 50 years of age was attacked with a burning in the throat, difficulty of swallowing, severe headache, and other symptoms belonging to this fatal disease. Domestic remedies were applied, but to no purpose. She was seen on the third day after the attack. There appeared ulcers and matter in the throat; fever, headache, loss of appetite, difficulty of swallowing, stiffness of the neck, weight about the stomach, anxiety, tightness about the heart, difficult breathing, hollow voice, much weakness, and tongue very brown.

A vomit was given, followed by a dose of Calomel and Salts. A mustard plaster was applied to the throat, gargles of the stronger kind ordered to be used, and her feet to be bathed in warm water. She appeared to be better after the vomit and physic had operated, but in forty-eight hours both were repeated, the gargles continued and sour drinks given; she was also permitted to smoke tobacco, having been in that habit. Her diet was light but nourishing; no cold water was allowed, and after the second physic her throat grew better, the fever disappeared and without any further prescription she recovered, she having been sick about eight days.

CASE No. 6.

A boy of about sixteen years, having been at a neighbor's where the Black Tongue prevailed, was attacked the next night. Paying but little attention to the symptoms, and having exposed himself in a shower of rain during the day, in the night he became delirious. When first seen by me, swelling had commenced in his throat, with the appearance of ulcers and offensive matter. There was, also, fever; an offensive breath, desire to vomit, inflamed eyes, pain in the stomach, headache, and difficulty in swallowing. His voice was changed, and his pulse extremely variable. A vomit was given, followed by Calomel and Salts. A blister was applied to the back of the neck, and gargles of Myrrh and Cayenne pepper used. The next night he again became delirious, and continued so three nights successively, perfectly rational through the day, though fearful of death. In forty-eight hours the emetic and physic were repeated, the gargles still continued, his feet bathed in warm water, and mustard plasters applied to the calves of the legs. The delirium then disappeared, but the ulcers in the throat appeared dangerous.— Therefore, another vomit was given, during the operation of which he perspired freely, which was encouraged by the administration of warm drinks.— From that time forward he grew better; the throat assumed its natural appearance; his fever disappeared; his appetite increased; his sleep was without interruption, and finally he recovered, having been sick about twelve days. His breath was very offensive until after the perspiration commenced. No cold water or strong diet was permitted in his case.

CASE No. 7.

A girl of about nine years of age, had been sick for about one week, having during that time used many domestic remedies to no purpose. When first seen, she could not talk above a whisper; her throat was covered by ashy-looking spots and matter; a greenish-looking water oozed from her nose; the fever was high; she complained much of pain in the stomach; her breath was offensive in the highest degree; a nervous twitching in her arms and feet was observed, with sunken eyes, a pale cadavarous countenance and skin hot and dry.

A strong emetic of Antimonial wine was given, and a blister applied to the back of the neck; after the emetic had operated and the blister drawn, a dose of Calomel was given, followed by salts, and gargles were used, of strong warm vinegar mixed with honey. The Calomel brought away a number of worms, after which the twitching of her limbs ceased. No cold water was permitted. The third day another vomit was given, and after that, during four days, repeated doses of Calomel, and upon the fifth day, in the morning, a dose of Salts, which produced four or five stools of a blackish color and very offensive smell. The gargling was, during all this time, continued once at least every four hours. A light sweat, together with a slight eruption on her arms, began to make their appearance, and from that time she commenced to mend. Her throat began to look better; the water ceased to run from her nose; her voice became more natural; her breath ceased to smell. She had been allowed to drink, daily, vinegar from pickled red beets, diluted with water, which she much relished. After the operation of the second vomit and physic, her fever disappeared, and in about eighteen days she was entirely well.

CASE No. 8.

A young woman of about twenty years of age; complained of much giddiness of the head; sick stomach; pain in the throat, especially when swallowing, with stiffness of the neck. Ulcers were found in the throat, and the tongue of a brown color, apparently very thickly coated; her voice was changed greatly; her breath smelled bad; there was also some fever.

A vomit was given, and strong gargles were used; in sixteen hours after the vomit, twenty grains of Calomel followed; four hours after, a table-spoon-full of Salts and a Mustard plaster upon the throat. The next day about half a dose of Calomel was given without any salts; the gargles were continued, upon the two following days a half dose of Calomel was given each day, and on the fourth day a small dose of Salts, which brought away much offensive, dark-colored matter, after which the giddiness of the head altogether disappeared, and her throat commenced to appear more clean, but a little red. Gargles of the milder kind were now ordered to be used, and a tea-spoon-full of Salts directed to be taken the next day; after which time she mended rapidly, and soon gained her former strength, being of a robust constitution. The drinking of cold water was prohibited.

Many more cases might be described, but these may

suffice as an illustration of the treatment prescribed in these pages; and all that is necessary to insure a favorable result is, to follow reasonable indications and apply immediate and effectual remedies. Then, and then only, the cure prescribed for this awful disease will prove itself to be infallible.

TO PURIFY THE AIR AND PREVENT THE INFECTION.

Take one quart of tar, one pint of rye whiskey and two ounces of finely powdered Gum Myrrh; mix all well together. Then put into an iron or earthen vessel some live coals, and on them pour three or four table-spoons-full of the above mixture, and smoke the house, particularly the chamber of the patient, which may be repeated three or four times during each day. This remedy, simple as it is, will purify the air and give considerable ease to the patient. If there exists in the patient any difficulty of breathing, or oppression, no additional uneasiness will be experienced because of this smoke. At least I have never heard a patient complain thereof; while it has effectually prevented the contagion from attacking those engaged as nurses, except in cases where the infection had been previously imparted. The rosin which oozes from wounds upon the pine tree might, perhaps, answer the same purpose where tar can not be had; and the smoking should be continued as long as any one about the house continues to be affected with the disease.

PRESCRIPTIONS ALLUDED TO IN THE FORE-GOING TREATMENT.

No. 1. *Vomit for persons of fourteen years and upwards.*

Take Ipecacuanha, from 15 to 20 grains; Tartar emetic, 2 grains; mix with about four table-spoons-full of hot water until perfectly dissolved. Give the patient two table-spoons-full, and in fifteen minutes after, let him drink a pint or half pint of warm water. It this be without effect, in fifteen minutes more give him another table-spoon full of the mixture, followed by more warm water. If vomiting is not produced after the second dose, give him another spoon-full of the mixture, followed by warm water. The more warm water he drinks the easier will be the operation.

No. 2. *A vomit for children from four to five years of age.*

Give the patient Antimonial wine, (from an apothecary or physician) from one to four tea-spoons-full, in warm water, every fifteen minutes, till the desired effect is produced. Let the doses be accompanied by repeated drinks of warm water, as above directed, and the quantity of the medicine regulated according to the age of the patient, (see table.)

No. 3. *Physic for adults of fourteen years and upwards.*

From 15 to 20 grains of Calomel, taken in honey, apple-butter, or molasses, followed in about six or eight hours by from a half ounce to an ounce of Salts.

No. 4. *Physic for children from one to fourteen years old.*

Take Calomel, the dose regulated according to age, (see table) followed in three or four hours by one or two tea-spoons-lull of Salts or Castor Oil.

No. 5. *Another, for the same.*

Take one ounce of Senna leaves, and a half ounce of

Manna; put it into a quart of water and boil down to a pint; which strain. Of this a person above fourteen years may take three table-spoons-full every two hours, until it operates. Children from two to fourteen years old, one or two table-spoons-full every four hours, as above. This physic is of a very mild nature, and, if prepared in the above manner, is seldom injurious, even when too freely used.

No. 6. *Another mild physic.*

Take an ounce of Salts, finely powdered, and mix thoroughly with a half ounce of Magnesia. Give an adult two table-spoons-full in sweet milk, or sage tea, every four hours until it begins to operate. A child may take from one to two tea-spoons-full every two hours, until it operates.

No. 7. *A mild acid drink.*

Take one ounce of Oil of Vitriol; (Oleum Vitrioli) mix with eight ounces of water and about three table-spoons-full of Brandy or Alcohol. Of this mixture drop about one hundred drops into a pint of water, which an adult patient may drink during one day. If under fourteen years, one fourth or one-half of the pint will do for one day. Vinegar in which red beets have been pickled, diluted with water, may answer in some cases in its stead; or sour cider vinegar, mixed with water, may be given more or less during the day, and when drink is asked for by the patient.

No. 8. *A strong gargle.*

Take Gum Myrrh, once ounce; powder it coarsely and add Cayenne pepper, one-fourth of an ounce; put both into one pint of French Brandy; let it stand in a warm place for two or three days, shaking it occasionally.—Then, in order to prepare it for gargling, take one tea-spoon-full of it to about one tea-spoon-full of warm water, or vinegar, and gargle with it every three or four

hours. If you want to make it stronger and more effectual, take two or three tea spoons-lull of it to a tea-cup-
full of strong warm vinegar.

No. 9. *A mild gargle for children.*

Take Blackberry juice, one tea-spoon-full; strong vinegar, one tea-cup-full, and three table-spoons-full of honey; mix it well; then put one table-spoon-full of the
mixture into one tea-cup-full of warm water, and gargle
with it. This is one of the mildest gargles that can be
procured.

No. 10. *For Injection.*

Take half a tea-cup-full of Sweet Oil, mix it with
about a pint of sweet milk, somewhat warm; this quantity will answer for an adult; for children the quantity may
be somewhat decreased. A syringe may be used for
administering it; if one can not be had a bladder with a
quill tied into it may answer for the same purpose.

No. 11. *A Liniment.*

Take Hartshorn, two ounces; Sweet Oil, two ounces;
shake them well together; then anoint the outside of the
neck three or four times a day, with about two tea spoons-
full of it at a time. Or a flannel rag may be made wet
with the mixture and laid on the throat; and in the course
of five or six hours it may be removed.

To prepare a Mustard Plaster.

Take yellow Mustard, ground or powdered, say two
table-spoons-full, and add to it a sufficient quantity of
strong vinegar to make it the consistence of mush; then
spread it upon a muslin or linen rag about the size of a
hand or less, (to be spread about one-fourth of an inch
in thickness,) and lay it on the throat or back of the neck.
When it has made the skin a good deal red, (which will
require, sometimes, only half an hour, othertimes, from

four to six hours,) take it off, grease a rag with a little sweet tallow or lard, and lay it on the parts, which will make them again easy. If it should have raised small blisters, a poultice of light bread and sweet milk must be applied, the blisters drawn and the water let out before a greased rag is put on; because, if this be neglected, the water in the blisters will produce irritation and soreness.

Directions for the drawing and attention of a Fly Blister.

Spread Spanish fly blister salve (which may be obtained of any apothecary or regular physician,) on a piece of coarse linen or soft leather about three inches long and four inches broad, for the back of the neck, or, if for the throat, about two and a half inches broad and four or five inches in length. Rub the parts to which this plaster is to be applied, with a woolen rag dipped in warm vinegar; then lay the blister on; let it lay some four or eight hours, when very likely it will have drawn a bladder, which must be opened on the lower part with a pair of scissors, making an incision of about one inch, taking care that the water which runs out does not touch any other parts of the flesh; for it is of such a corroding nature, sometimes, as to produce a blister wherever it touches. When thus opened, a poultice of soft light bread boiled in sweet milk, to the consistence or thickness of mush, must be applied until the water ceases to run from the wound; and renewed every four or six hours, when a small rag, greased with sweet oil, fresh lard or butter, laid on about once a day will heal it. If a little sweet cream be applied to the sides of each poultice it will prevent the poultice from adhering to the skin when about to be removed. The more a blister is poulticed, the better for the patient. If after the blister has laid on for the time specified, there should be small white blisters visible, like watery pimples, about the size of a pea, the plaster may be removed, and a poultice of light bread and sweet milk applied; or a cabbage leaf scalded with boiling water, or wilted by the fire, will answer, permitting either to lay on about one hour.— This will have drawn the bladder up, which must be opened and treated as before stated. A blister once used upon a patient afflicted with this disease, must never be applied to any one else; for it has been observed, in more than one case, to infect others with the same disease.— This may seem strange, but it is nevertheless so, and deserves the attention of practising physicians. The blister ought to be burnt, or, if used again, let it be used by the same person.

It has happened some times that the person on whom a blister is drawn, becomes affected with a kind of strangury, or difficulty of voiding urine, attended with pain in the parts. This need not produce uneasiness or unnecessary fear. If it should take place, let the patient drink flaxseed tea, or tea made of parsley root, and apply a warm poultice to the lower parts of the stomach, such as hops boiled in water, or even rags dipped in warm water. They must, however, be renewed when they begin to get cold, and discontinued when the difficulty and pain ceases.

Table of the Doses for Different Ages, Intended as a Guide to the Foregoing Treatment.

DOSES.	Children 1 month old.	3 months old.	6 months old.	1 year old.	4 years old.	8 years old.	14 years old.	Adults.
Dose of Calomel for physic.	1 1-2 grain.	2 1-2 grains.	3 grains.	4 grains.	6 grains.	10 grains.	15 grains.	20 to 25 grs., if a male; 15 to 20 grs., if a female.
Antimonial Wine as a vomit.	6 drops every 10 min. until effectual.	12 drops, repeated in 10 minutes.	18 grains.	A small tea-spoonful, re-peated in 15 minutes.	A tea-spoonful, repeated in 10 min., un-til effectual.	2 tea-spoons-full, repeat-ed in 10 min-utes.	1 table-spoon-ful every 15 min., until effectual.*	2 table-spoonsfull in 10 min., un-til effectual.*
Dose of Salts to follow the Calomel.	1-2 teaspoon-ful, disolved in tea or wa-ter.	A tea-spoon-ful, repeated in 12 hours if necessary.	A good tea-spoonful.	1 1-2 tea-spoons-full.	2 tea-spoons-full.	3 tea-spoons-full	1 table spoonful.	2 table spoons-full, and more if necessary.
Dose of Castor Oil.	1-2 teaspoon-ful every six hours, until it operates.	A small tea-spoon-ful.	1 good tea-spoonful.	1 1-2 tea-spoons-full.	2 tea-spoons-full.	1 tablespoon-ful.	1 1-2 table-spoons-full.	From 2 to 3 table-spoons-full.

*In each case warm water to be given freely after the wine.

The Measles commonly are of so mild a nature that, with ordinary care, but few children die with them, unless there already exists a complaint of the breast, or hereditary disposition to Consumption.—But there are examples on record of Measles having existed in different places which put an end to the lives of all attacked. From this cause, I suppose, the ancient Latins gave that disease the name of Morbilli, or the little Plague; and of this description were the Measles which existed in Stockholm in 1713, where so many persons died. A more malignant description of Measles existed in Vienna in the year 1732; most of the patients having died with mortification in the throat on the third or fourth day. In London the Measles prevailed in 1672 to such a fatal extent that the deaths numbered three hundred per week. The Measles which existed in Edinburgh, in Scotland, was of so mild a nature, that only about every twelfth patient died. According to Morton's account, there died, in 1672, in London, three thousand six hundred persons in three months with the Measles; and in the year 1742, there died nine hundred and eighty-one in the same place. The Measles which then prevailed were no doubt of a malignant character.

The Measles most always exist epidemically, and the contagion is spread in the same manner as that of the Small Pox. They have consequently their own peculiar poison, which hardly ever exists in the air,

A14

but is carried about and scattered over a country by
the people and their clothing; therefore, it is possible
to escape them, just as well as the Small Pox, if care
is taken not to go where the Measles are. Nor is it
possible that a person should be twice afflicted with
the Measles if properly cured upon the first attack.—
However, in cases of improper treatment, when they
have been imperfectly cured, a return is not at all impossible. An example of this kind is mentioned by
Dr. Home in his " Medical Facts and Experiments,"
page 250. Dr. Haarrman and Dr. De Haen say it is
possible to have the Measles the second time, but they,
and others who maintain the same idea, have against
them a majority of physicians, who are of a contrary
opinion, to wit, that no one who has had the real
Measles once, and been actually cured, will be ever
after afflicted with them again. Dr. Rosenstein says
he has never seen it once during a practice of forty-
four years.

No age or sex is exempt from the attacks of this
complaint, and the aged man and the infant are equal-
ly liable. It is true that in some places, where the
Measles were prevailing, some persons did not get
them, remaining free from them during their existence; it may also be that in every hundred persons,
four or five will never get them. As with the Small
Pox, so it may be with the Measles; but nothing can
be said of this with certainty. It is, and will remain
a supposition, upon which no foundation of a gene-
ral rule can be laid.

Commonly, the Measles will attack children, but
very old people have taken them too, while there are

examples on record of childfen being born with them.
But they never come through fear or fright. When
the Measles commence in a place, or neighborhood,
they generally continue so long as there are any left
who have never had them, or until the healthy persons, through fear, are induced to shun all intercourse
with those who are afflicted with them, which should
be especially practised if the Measles are of a malignant nature. It is generally supposed that the Small
Pox after six weeks loses its infective power in a person affected by it, provided he then changes his clothing. According to this, the patients under the Measles should not be bound on a quarntine of that length;
because the infective power of the Measles, it is said,
will not last as long as that of the Small Pox.

A return of the Measles is supposed to be frequent
by the unlearned classes of people, but the skilful
physician will usually find the disease to be either
Chicken Pox, Scarlet Fever, or some other eruptive
fever, the distinction between which the ignorant are
unable to make.

SYMPTOMS.

If, during the prevalence of the Measles, there appears a dry cough, frequent sneezing, running of water from the eyes and nose, which appears warm to
the person affected, with more or less fever, then beyond a doubt he is about to be attacked by the Measles. These signs are always present with the Measles; but in an epidemic of Measles it may happen
that the symptoms are somewhat changed, and require an experienced, penetrating and discerning judgment to recognise them. Generally, they commence

with a feeling of coldness, followed by a hot stage
of uncertain duration. This heat increases upon the
second day, and there appears a dry cough; running,
watery eyes, and frequent sneezing. If the cough is
frequent and violent, the eyes run less, and the sneezing is not so frequent; and so on the contrary, if the
cough is light and seldom, the eyes will run more,
and the sneezing be more frequent. Besides this the
face looks somewhat bloated, the eyelids begin to
swell, and are somewhat difficult to open, with aversion to light; the patient complains of weakness, heaviness of the head; a feeling of weight on the breast, pain
in the throat and small of the back. An inclination to
vomit, or actual vomiting comes on, together with a
loathing of food; great thirst; a coated, whiteish-look-
ing tongue; cholic, and a loose state of the bowels;
bleeding of the nose and delirium, and, in some cases,
passing convulsive fits. All these are attended by
great inclination to sleep, and a continued high fever,
which, however, is not found in all cases.

About the fourth day there appear, in great num-
bers, on the face, small red spots, which on the first
day are a little elevated above the skin. In this con-
sists the grand distinction between the Measles and
the Scarlet Fever. On the second day after appearing, these spots are even with the skin, and appear
in broad red spots; their shape is not always round,
but they may be of all kinds of shapes and forms;
they increase gradually in number and size, and appear by degrees, on the neck, breast, arms, back, legs,
and all over the body. But on their first appearance
they appear as even red spots.

These symptoms do not decrease in violence or strength through the eruption, as in the Small Pox. The vomiting only ceases in some cases. On the contrary, the symptoms increase in violence, especially the fever, the weight on the breast, the difficulty of breathing, the cough, the weakness and the watering of the eyes; together with the disposition to sleep, and loathing of all food.

On the sixth or seventh day the skin on the face and forehead begins to feel a little rough; the spots thereon decrease in number, and dry off; while those on other parts of the body are larger and more red. On the eighth day there is scarcely one of them to be seen on the whole body; on the ninth day they altogether disappear. But instead of these spots, it will be observed that the skin peals off in small, thin scales; or that the surface of the body appears as if sprinkled over with flour; now, persons generally suppose that all danger is over; but at this time it often happens that fever returns stronger than before; the difficulty of breathing increases, and the cough is so hard and troublesome, that the patient finds no rest. Frequently there now appears a diahrroea, which proves suddenly beneficial, but which, if too severe, will weaken the patient, and if it continues, may induce lingering fever, or consumption, and should be attended to carefully. Should no diarrhœa appear at this period the patient will nevertheless do well if a moderate perspiration follows, or should be induced. A repeated bleeding of the nose will remove the headache and heaviness of the head, together with the soreness of the eyes, neck, or throat. If only the proper evacuations, hereafter mentioned; are carefully attended to, there will be no cause to fear the above sad and dangerous consequences.

But if it should happen that the fever continues, together with the cough, and the breathing grows more difficult, with hot breath, and there appears a redness of the cheeks, these are bad symptoms, and indicate a disposition to inflamation of the lungs. If the fever continues and a violent pain in the side appears, then the patient certainly is in great danger; also, if the throat becomes inflamed and swelled so_ that the drawing of breath is difficult and the swallowing painful. Should the fever decrease, but still daily show itself, accompanied by difficult breathing, or shortness of breath, emaciation of the patient, and the coughing up of much matter, it may be considered as a sign of an already formed ulcer or sore in the lungs.

If the Measles strike in too soon, in consequence of which the patient becomes delirious, then is he also in great danger. Very red or pale looking spots, also indicate approaching danger. Also, Measles that break out at an earlier or later period than above stated, are more or less dangerous.

In some epidemics the Measles are, in many children, of so mild a nature that the eruption appears before they complain of any sickness whatever. Pregnant women and women in child-bed, are in great danger with the Measles, and require very careful attention. Persons having a weak breast, or a disposition to hæmorrhage, are always in more danger and suffer more through the cough than others. Convulsion fits are to be feared, if the patient, during the first stage of the Measles, sweats a good deal and passes little or no urine. The excitement of the mind in females, by anger or fear, is accompanied with great danger to the child if it has the Measles, and is allowed to suck at that time.

Small Pox and Measles sometimes exist in a neighborhood at the same time. But it is seldom that a person has Small Pox and Measles at the same time, although Dr. Bergius mentions some examples of that kind.

The cause of the Measles is no other than the Measle poison, which mixes itself with the blood, and produces or creates an irritation. The troublesome cough is produced from a part of the poison being drawn into the lungs through the breath, and having there produced the same kind of an eruption inwardly as appears externally, hindering, in a measure, the excreation of the same. Externally the eruption falls off in scales, or like flour; this happens in the lungs, also, but they being always moist, the process is slower. In the meantime they contain something which continually irritates the patient to cough, and in no other manner can it be brought away, except by coughing. If what is coughed up grows harder, or of a more solid nature, then it will so much easier carry along with it the above mentioned scales or flour-like matter. That this is so, may be plainly seen by attentively reading Dr. Homes' description of the progress of the Measles, in cases produced by him by innoculation, as in the Small Pox. The most of them had no cough at all, but some few had a slight cough, which was of so mild a nature that no attention was

paid to it. It will be observed, from what has been
said, that while the Small Pox has four different stages,
the Measles have but three.

The first (Stadium contagii) commences with the
beginning of the sickness, and ends when the Measles
appear, or break out.

The second (Stadium eruptionis) commences from
the time of the eruption, and ends when it begins to
peal off in scales or like fine powder.

The third (Stadium exarescentiæ) commences with
the sixth and seventh day, and ends with the eighth
and ninth, when the Measles will have disappeared.

We will consider each of them separate, and show
some of the attention which is, more or less, necessary during the different stages of the Measles.

THE FIRST STAGE.—If the existing Measles are of
a mild character, and the patient has otherwise no
breast complaint, there will be seldom any thing else
necessary than good nursing. The nursing is somewhat similar to that required in the Small Pox, only
that the patient requires more warm drink, more bed-
clothes, and a warmer bed-room. The patient ought
not to eat or drink any thing sour, on account of the
troublesome cough. The poison of the Measles is
more subtle than in the Small Pox, and can therefore
far easier go inward again, in consequence of which
the patient with the Measles requires greater care than
with the Small Pox. The room where the patient
lays ought not to be crowed; only those engaged in
nursing should be allowed to be with him; also, there
ought to be little light in the room during the night.

If the Measles which exist in a neighborhood are of a very malignant character, then it is always necessary.

First, to bleed; regulating the quantity of blood taken according to the age and constitution of the patient. There might be many reasons given to show the necessity of this, but I only quote the celebrated Dr. Mead, who always bled his patients in the Measles, that an inflamation of the lungs might be prevented. The blood was always coated with a thick hide of bad-looking matter, when suffered to get cold.— He also says that under this treatment he never lost a patient. Dr. Rosenstein agrees with him in this matter, and says it is absolutely necessary, if there are signs of an inflamamatory state of the blood and system.

Secondly, it is necessary that the patient either take a vomit or a physic, according to circumstances. If there is an inclination to vomit, an unclean looking tongue, with a bitter taste in the mouth, and giddiness and headache, then the vomiting ought to be encouraged. To this end the patient may drink warm water, or get from the apothecary three grains of Ipecacuanha, which mix thoroughly with eighteen grains of loaf sugar, and divide into three equal parts. One of these is a dose for a child of about two or three years old, and may be taken in a little warm tea. If it does not vomit in fifteen minutes, give another; if without effect, in fifteen minutes give the third powder, after which certainly vomiting will follow.

If none of the aforementioned indications are present, but the stomach of the patient appears bloated, with a rumbling noise in the bowels and an inclination to stool, but without a passage, then a mild laxative is necessary, which may be Castor Oil or Salts· If attention is paid to the timely evacuations of the stomach and bowels before the Measles break out, it will prevent many other difficulties during the further progress of the disease; and especially, it will render the diarrhœa, which generally comes on the eighth or ninth day, of a mild nature and healing consequence.

If the patient should in the beginning, be troubled with pain in the stomach and diarrhœa, he must at any rate make use of a mild laxative, which may consist of a light dose of Rhubarb, which medicine has a tendency to take off the cause of the irritation of the bowels and stomach, and also, by degrees, stop the diarrhoea.

Thirdly:—After this the patient may make use of the following means, more or less; first, a little lighter bed covering; second, a little less heat in the room, taking care not to catch cold; third, milk-warm teas, of sage, catnip, or mint..

Care must also be taken of the eyes, keeping them from the light, and washing occasionally with a little good rosewater, which will wash away the sharp water and prevent the eyes from becoming inflamed.

If the nose should bleed, it ought not to be suppressed suddenly, for the bleeding will have a tendency to remove the headache and delirium; but if it should continue too long, so that the face grows pale and the hands and feet get cold, or until the patient begins to complain of an inclination to vomit, then it ought to be immediately stopped, which may be done as follows. Rub a little alum in the white of an egg until the egg forms in lumps; then take a little cotton, dipped in this substance, and insert in the nostril as far as it can be got. It may be left in for a day or two.

The cough is always the greatest trouble in the Measles, for which a good remedy may be found in tea of elder blossoms, mixed with about a fifth part of sweet milk and sweetened with a little sugar or molasses A good addition to this will be a little liquorice dissolved in the tea. The cough is very difficult and troublesome, but seldom dangerous until after the Measles are gone. If the throat should have an appearance as if getting sore, a mild gargle of sage tea, sweetened with honey, should be used; or flaxseed tea may answer the same end. Externally, a Mustard plaster may be applied until the skin becomes somewhat reddened.

THE SECOND STAGE.—When the fourth day comes round, the patient should remain as quiet as possible, for now a very mild perspiration only is to be desired Experience has shown that the Measles then will come out well and leave free the interior of the body. He may then, if deemed necessary, take a mild vomit, but especially warm drinks are to be recommended, which are necessary, even when Measles have come out well. After the eruption appears, the color of it deserves our attention next; and also whether it continues three days or not, and whether it gradually disappears in the same order as it appeared. If the color be very red, cooling vegetable drink should be freely given; but if only in some places red and in others pale, a little warm tea of common Sheep Saffron may be given, or a dose or two of Sweet Spirits of Nitre, regulated according to age, is an excellent remedy at this stage, which will answer also if the Measles should strike in again too early. Or the patient may freely use tea of elder blossoms, and if he is delirious lay a Spanish fly blister upon the back of his neck and permit it to draw effectually. Also, Mustard plasters may be applied to the calves of the legs If by these means the Measles appear again, then there is no need of fear of danger, but it is advisable, however, to keep the patient secure from cold, anger, fright, ect., so that the Measles may not strike in again.

The patient will generally in this stage be very restless, and requires, therefore, so much more care and attention from those who have him in charge.

The Third Stage.—This is the most dangerous period, which soon determines the fate of the patient. The closest attention to the patient is therefore highly necessary. If it is found that the skin is soft, and the pulse decreasing in strength, then a mild perspiration or good sweat may be expected, during which the fever will disappear. Some lukewarm drink may be given during the perspiration. But if the perspiration or sweat does not come on, and there is no rumbling noise in the bowels, nor a bloated state of the stomach, then warm drinks, such as mint or pennyroyal tea, are highly necessary, in order to bring perspiration, taking care not to give more than is necessary for that purpose. But if the skin should be dry, and the patient complain of ague in the stomach, together with a rumbling in the bowels, then diarrhœa may be expected, which generally comes on suddenly, producing perhaps ten or twelve stools in a very short time. If this gives relief, so that the cough grows less, the eyes look livelier, the patient can move with less difficulty, and the bloated state of the stomach disappears, then the diarrhœa will be followed by good consequences, and must not be checked too soon. If it should be attended by much pain, which will not cease upon applying a warm poultice to the stomach, the patient may take a small dose of Rhubarb, according to his age, and lay upon the stomach a plaster composed as follows: A quarter of an ounce of Theriac, half a drachm of Nutmeg oil, and three drops of Oil of Caraway; which mix carefully and spread upon a piece of leather, to be applied to the stomach. But if the diarrhoea should become too violent and continue too long, it must then be checked, which may be done in different ways; either by some scorched flour, stirred in sweet milk and given to the patient, or by a powder composed of four parts of Camphor finely powdered, and one part Opium, (say four grains of Camphor, and one grain, or a half grain of Opium.) If the disease does not yield to this treatment and the fever increases, with a continuance of the cough, difficulty of breathing, the breath feels hot and there is a redness of the cheeks, then a new fever is forming, which is called peripneumonia or inflamation of the lungs.

This is very dangerous. The patient should be bled immediately, and in the same arm or side where the reddest cheek is; after which lay a Spanish fly blister between the shoulders, and when it has drawn, another one on the side from which the blood has been taken. If a difficulty of voiding urine, or much pain in the parts, should come on, a little flaxseed tea will soon remove it. If these means somewhat ease the difficulty of breathing, then warm pennyroyal tea may be given in order to produce a light sweat. If the patient after that commences to cough up a yellowish matter, tinged with blood, then there is some hope of his recovery, and acid drinks may be given, such as Cream of Tartar.

Should he be costive at this time, an injection morning and evening may serve a good purpose. But if the patient should have a violent pain in the side instead of the above mentioned symptoms, and the fever be increasing, blood should be taken from the arm of the same side, and a Spanish fly blister laid on the place where the pain is felt. After it has drawn give warm drinks freely; but as soon as the coughing up of matter commences, then the bleeding ought not to be repeated, neither the sweating too much encouraged, because it may have a tendency to stop the cough, which at present is of great benefit to the patient in bringing away the bad matter contained or gathered in the lungs.

If the patient will not permit a blister to be put on, then a Mustard plaster may perhaps answer the same end; or, rub the following composed oil upon the side in which the pain is felt: Take Oil of Flaxseed, or Sweet Almonds, two ounces; dissolve in it half an ounce of Camphor, with which anoint the side three or four times a day. Or blood may be drawn from the side by cupping; but if nothing of that kind can be had, a half loaf of bread, fresh from the oven, laid on as hot as it can be endured, will answer some-times just as well. But it may happen that as the fever decreases it reappears every afternoon, together with a hoarseness and shortness of breath, and cough-ing up of much matter; then the patient should use a good deal of milk, especially if he seems to fall away in flesh; or the following drink may be used: Boil one ounce of Peruvian bark in one quart of water for about fifteen minutes; then strain it, and add to it one quart of sweet milk; drink one quart of it during one day, if the patient be an adult; for children, give less. This drink will be of great benefit, if the evacuations of the stomach and bowels have been well attended to before using it.

The eyes, also, in the third stage of the Measles, are generally red and may become very troublesome if not taken care of. It has been directed before to wash them with rosewater, but if this has not been sufficient to allay the inflammation, there may be some leaches applied to the temples or eyelids; or, a small Spanish fly blister may be laid on each temple, and well drawn, after which mild laxative medicine should be administered, such as Castor Oil or Salts; which, according to his strength, may be repeated once or twice; or one of the following poultices may be laid over the eyes: Take the white of an egg, beat it up with alum until it becomes thick; then spread a linen rag and apply it—to be renewed in about six hours. Or you may take raw potatoes, scraped finely and spread upon a rag; lay it on and renew it every two or three hours. Or you may apply a poultice made of light bread and sweet milk, and renew it every six hours. Or you may take a red winter apple, roast it under hot ashes, then take the seed out and mash it up, and mix under it about five grains of finely powdered Camphor; spread a poultice of it and lay it on, renewing it every six hours. Camphor will not powder well, except you drop on it a few drops of Sulphuric Æther; when that cannot be had and the powdered Camphor is only intended for external use, a little good rye whiskey may then be dropped on it, which will answer sufficiently well for external use.

Enough has been said to enable a discerning mind to form an idea of the treatment necessary for a favorable result in this disease; it is true, circumstances happen which would require some alterations, but that will depend upon so many different causes, that it will be difficult to lay down or prescribe a treatment for so many supposed cases. Neither would it answer here, for it would only perplex the minds of some, who would not be able to distinguish the right remedy from the wrong one, having had little or no experience in that line of business. Therefore, let them make good use of what has been laid down, follow reasonable indications, apply suitable remedies, and the Measles will be very easy to manage, if good care is taken.

A SHORT TREATISE ON THE SCARLET FEVER.—[SCARLATINA.]

This is a fever accompanied by a nearly scarlet eruption, from which, perhaps, the complaint derives its name. Children are oftener attacked with it than adults. This fever makes its appearance seldom, yet is not confined to any particular season of the year, but may appear at all seasons. It bears some resemblance to the Measles, and also the Putrid Sore Throat, and the (so called) Wild Fire; but the whole progress of the disease and the bad consequences which sometimes follow it, go to show plainly that the disease deserves an exclusive title of distinction, and a careful treatment.

It generally commences with a soreness of the throat, together with a weakness and increased sensibility of the whole body. After ten or twelve hours there appears a sickness of the stomach, a vomiting of bad matter, mixed more or less with gall, shivering, headache, and a great inclination to sleep on the first day; sometimes the soreness and swelling of the throat will increase very rapidly; when the patient awakes from a sleep, he will be very restless and appear very anxious and fretful, having a difficulty of breathing, and a short heavy breath. It is seldom that convulsive fits will make their appearance.

In some the eruption will, after the foregoing symptoms have appeared, break out and show itself on the second or third day, in small red spots. They appear first in the face, and on the neck; then on the

breast, stomach, feet, legs, and nearly the whole body.
The eruption will occupy, in most cases, from twenty-four to thirty-six hours, and sometimes longer,
spreading gradually; and if the redness of the face begins somewhat to diminish, then the feet and legs will
look so much more inflamed. This eruption is not
in the least elevated above the skin; but it will happen that the part of the body which looks the reddest will seem somewhat thicker and rather swelled
than the rest, but which will disappear when the redness goes away. If the finger is pressed hard it will
look white, but soon it will regain its former red
color when withdrawn.

Until the end of the fourth day the swelling will,
in most cases, be somewhat difficult, and it will also
be noticed that the speaking is difficult, and apparently through the nose; after the fourth day more or less
hoarseness shows itself, and some commence to cough
up much matter and corruption. By gargling the
throat, the difficulty of swallowing will be greatly
removed, the eyes will look more lively, and the patient will be in better humour.

On the same day it will happen, sometimes, that
there will come on four, five, or six thin stools suddenly, which give, at times, great relief. Some have
a bleeding of the nose on or about the end of the fifth
day, which will also tend to enliven the patient; others
will get it on the seventh day or later, but also in a
light manner.

The heat and the fever, which has been tolerable
high, especially in the afternoon and towards evening,
will now generally commence to decrease and get

milder, but will seldom finally disappear until the seventh day.

Delirium, if it does happen, will generally happen towards the evening of the third or fourth day, but is not of much consequence, if it only disappears in the hours when the fever is not too high, and is somewhat lessened.

The pulse is more or less frequent; in some very strong; in others weak; and they will be harder affected than others.

The stools will seldom operate themselves, except on the mentioned day. If a sweat takes place it will mostly happen on the night of the fifth day; seldom before that time.

There is generally not so much spitting as in other sore throats, neither so much sneezing as in the measles, if any at all; the nose appears dry inwardly; the eyes do not run; the urine sometimes passes with difficulty, but is not so red as might be expected on account of the great heat. It will be seldom mixed with blood, though some writers have recorded examples of it.

Hardly any will be troubled with a cough until the throat begins to loosen, and then the coughing will be beneficial to the patient.

The patient complains mostly of soreness of the throat, the heat of the skin and the thirst accompanying it. On the fifth day the redness of the face, and upon the next day, the redness of the body, will gradually diminish, so that on the eighth day little or none will be seen.

On the sixth or seventh day some have observed in some patients, especially behind the ears and upon the neck, feet, and hands, small pale dry blisters; they . gradually spread, and then commences the pealing off of the thin skin over the whole body. This pealing off, in some cases, progresses rapidly; in others it takes from two to three weeks, particularly if the eruption has been great. Dr. Plenciz has observed that some cases had no pealing off of the skin at all.

With the eighth and ninth day the disease will, generally, apparently disappear; but it has been observed, that patients who exposed themselves to the air before the ninth day, were seized with a dropsy of the skin, or gathering of water under the hide, in which condition they voided an ashy, grey-looking urine, with a sediment of the same color. After the ninth day, the patient generally ceases to complain, gets a good appetite and begins to rest well. But the main thing now depends on not feeling too secure; for from exposure, or a neglect to stay in the room and take a mild laxative occasionally, or observe a mild diet, the patient may be afflicted with a swelling of the glands, something like the mumps, or perhaps of the whole body; a fever will come on again, together with anxiety, restlessness, oppression and shortness of breath; the urine then will only pass sparingly and sometimes bloody. At this period, that is, from the ninth to the tenth day, many patients loose their lives; not from the Scarlet Fever, but from the consequences of their own carelessness. I will here insert some of the observations of Dr. Plenciz:

1, Such a dropsy may follow sometimes, at any rate, especially if there has been much of an eruption, but that is no absolute consequence belonging to the disease.

2, That the swelling was generally greatest in those upon whom there had been much pealing off of the skin; but a few cases have happened in which there was much watery swelling and scarcely any pealing off of the skin.

3, That children are more subject to it than adult persons.

4, That it happened to a greater extent in the winter than in the summer; and especially in those exposed to the air during and between the ninth and twentieth days.

5, That more will die in this period than during the eruption; on account of carelessness.

6, That it may be prevented altogether by keeping the patient in the room, moderately warm, and using every second or third day a mild laxative, with moderation in eating and drinking.

I have thus far partially described the symptoms and progress of this disease; and it may be perhaps just to say, that the Scarlet Fever as far as is known, exists epidemically; but the opinion is generally prevalent, that no one will be twice afflicted with it. It will affect different persons of different constitutions in different ways, according as they are more or less susceptible to the poison and the subsequent infection of it.

By carefully reading the foregoing description, the Scarlet Fever will be easy to distinguish from other diseases, particularly when it is known to be in the neighborhood. It is true it has, in the beginning, nearly all the symptoms of other eruptive fevers; but if the patient has had the Small Pox already, there is no need of fear from it; neither if the left eye does not run, or water, and the eyes feel not hot, there will be no need of looking for the Small Pox; and if there is no dry cough or frequent sneezing, and no running of a hot water out of the eyes, there need be no expectation or fear of the Measles. After the eruption is once out, it is not easy to make a mistake then.— Altogether, the progress of the Scarlet Fever and its accompanying incidents, plainly show that it is a particular disease, separate altogether from other eruptive fevers, for,

1st., In the Small Pox, the eruption stands over the skin and is soon changed to matter and suppuration, but in the Scarlet Fever the spots are level, and not at all elevated above the skin.

2nd, In the Measles the eruption is not so red, and on the first day it is somewhat elevated above the skin in the face, the eyes run a kind of hot water, the sneezing is continued, the skin peals off more like flour, the scales not being so large as in Scarlet Fever. Besides this, the fever in the latter disease nearly disappears on the eighth day, while in the Measles, on the eighth or ninth day the fever is higher, the breathing more difficult and the cough more troublesome. Also, the soreness of the throat is not so great in other eruptive fevers as in the Scarlet Fever, and the small, pale empty bladders behind the ears and on the hands, feet, or neck, with which the pealing off often commences, are not observed in other eruptive fevers. The cause of Scarlet Fever is just as little known as the cause of the Small Pox and Measles; but it is known that the disease is contagious.

That the skin is somewhat inflamed in this disease is not difficult to see, for to inflamation belong redness, heat, pain, and swelling; but the inflamation here is not of such a nature as to produce suppuration or the formation of matter, but only causes the external skin to separate from the internal and fall off in consequence; the inflamation of the throat must he of the same nature as the inflamation of the skin, for it neither causes suppuration, but falls off in like manner, though carelessness brings on mortification.— Dr. Plenciz has shown in his observations on Scarlet Fever, that such pealing off of the skin in the throat actually took place.

The Scarlet Fever is sometimes so mild that only good nursing is needed; at other times so violent and malignant as to prove fatal on the first or second day.

It is generally called a good sign, if the eruption appears gradually and not before the third day; and if the fever grows less after the eruption has appeared, it is also a favorable symptom.

Great inflamation in the throat and difficulty in swallowing; great heat of the skin; a quick but weak pulse; difficult heavy breathing; weakness and high fever; great inclination to sleep, or no sleep at all; great delirium, preceded by painful headache; restlessness, and tossing in the bed, and picking with the fingers in the air, are dangerous symptoms.

If the eruption should appear irregularly, and in places looking more or less red, then there may follow a frightful delirium, which will bring on death, preceded, sometimes, by a deadness of one side of the body; if it should then happen that a kind of bloody matter runs out of the ears, or from one ear only, there is some cause to hope for the better. In the time of the breaking out of the eruption, some patients spit away bloody-looking matter, and also pass bloody urine, followed by more or less swelling of the body afterwards.

If after a severe attack of the fever, the patient loses his appetite, looks pale, complains of weakness and can not pass his urine freely, he is in danger of dropsy, and speedy aid is necessary.

The cure is nearly similar to that prescribed in the first period of the Measles. As a drink, water first boiled and then mixed with about one-third of sweet milk, is advisable, and the patient should not, under the most favorable circumstances, leave his room under three weeks.

When the fever is violent, the patient, if an adult, should be bled, which may perhaps be necessary to repeat in eight or twelve hours; for children, cupping of the back of the neck and breast may answer. If there is much sickness of the stomach, accompanied by vomiting, it should be encouraged by giving warm water, or a vomit may be given with good effect.— When the vomiting has ceased; which sometimes happens soon, it is generally followed by a stool; but if this should not happen, and the stomach is somewhat bloated, a mild laxative should be given; such as Castor Oil, Salts, or Rhubarb. If the eruption is expected to appear soon, an injection of Sweet Oil and sweet milk may be administered instead of the laxative, which injection may be given once a day or every other day.

The throat also requires peculiar attention; to which end a handful of the dried blossoms of hollow haws, mixed with two table-spoonsful of bruised flaxseed, boiled together to a thick mush with sweet milk, may be applied as a poultice to the throat, and renewed two or three times; or a mustard plaster may be applied instead of the above. A gargle may also be used, composed of sage tea in which figs have been boiled, with which the patient should gargle his throat five or six times a day. The nostrils may be moistened with a little sweet milk; if the nose appears very dry and stopped up, a rag dipped in vinegar in which elder blossoms have been boiled, may be laid upon the breast, that the steam may pass to the patient's nose. If all this will give no relief, a small Spanish fly blister may be laid behind the ear until effectually drawn.

If the patient coughs up lumps of slime it is a favorable indication, and the neck and throat should then be well covered, and gargles freely used with cooling drinks. If bleeding of the nose comes on, it may be stopped as directed in the treatment of Measles.

In case of high fever and delirium upon the evening of the first day, which delirium ceases when the fever decreases, it is only necessary to give such medicines as tend to allay the fever as before mentioned. But if the delirium returns on the sixth, seventh or following days, then it is dangerous and requires attention; if an adult, bleeding may be used and a Spanish fly blister laid on the back of the neck; if a child, injections may be given and mustard plasters laid on the calves of the legs. On the fourth and fifth day, tea of elder blossoms may be freely given, for before that time it will be useless to give any thing to encourage perspiration, as the skin can not be moist as long as it is inflamed. It is not advisable to give strong medicines or teas to produce sweating, but when a perspiration takes place, it should be carefully attended to.

When the fever and redness of skin disappears, and

the patient recovers his appetite, his stomach should be rubbed morning and evening with a woolen rag smoked with Juniper berries, a mild laxative be given every two or three days and the utmost care taken in his diet.

If symptoms of dropsy should appear, let the patient freely drink tea of roasted Juniper berries, or flaxseed, parsley root, ect., and continue the laxatives until all appearance of the disease is gone. Then the body of the patient may be washed with warm wine or brandy once or twice a day, which will tend to revive his strength.

By careful attention during the progress of this disease, and the application of such means as have been mentioned, the most favorable results may be confidently expected.

RECEIPTS OF GREAT VALUE.

For the Dropsy, or Watery Swelling of the Legs, Arms and Body.

Dropsy is known by a swelling of the feet and legs, sometimes of the arms and body, upon which a mark or hollow is left after a pressure by the finger. The receipt here prescribed is simple, but worthy of confidence, as it has been the means of saving many lives. Its use should be continued three or four weeks, or as many months, if necessary.

Take two handsfull of the inside of dogwood bark, boil it in half a gallon of strong vinegar about half an hour; then put into it thirty-five or forty old rusty iron nails, and boil about twenty minutes longer, which will make it look as black as ink; then take it off, strain it, let it cool and settle, when it is fit for

use. After a physic has been taken, of salts or castor oil, give the patient, if he be an adult, half a tea-
cupful three times a day; if over twenty years old,
one small teacup-ful three times a day; a patient from
five to fourteen years old may take from three to four
tablespoons-full three times a day; from two to five
years old, from one to two tablespoons-full three
times a day, is sufficient.

The first four doses may produce sickness and
vomiting, but after that no inconvenience will be felt.
The water will pass off in the ordinary manner in a
surprising quantity. Parsley root tea may be given,
or flaxseed tea, during the use of the medicine.

ANOTHER FOR THE SAME DISEASE.

Take one ouce of Saltpetre, and dissolve it in half
a gallon of water. After a physic has been taken, the
dose for an adult over twenty years of age is, a tea-
cupful twice a day; from five to ten years old, two
tablespoonsful three times a day. Flax seed tea or
parsley-root tea should also be given. This is a safe
and speedy cure, if the patient is otherwise healthy.
The use of it should be continued three or four weeks,
or longer if necessary.

ANOTHER FOR THE SAME.

Take the inner bark of what is called White Elder,
from the first joint above the ground down to the
ground, pealed downward, of which put one good
handful into one quart of water; boil it down to one
pint, strain and drink of it one pint per day for three
days. Then take the inner bark of the root of the
same elder, (pealed downward also) two good handsful, and put it into one quart of water; boil it down

to one pint, then strain and take half a tea-cupful every four hours, until it operates freely on the bowels. This will occupy four days; after which it should be continued in the same manner for twelve days more; that is to say, the tea of the bark of the stem is to be used for three days, and the fourth day, the bark of the root is to be used in tea as a physic, and so on alternating. Children under fourteen years should take a lesser quantity, in proportion to their age.— Tea of parsley or flaxseed may also be used.

For BALDNESS OF THE HEAD, AND FALLING OUT OF THE HAIR.

This receipt has been kept very secret in Europe during many years. Take sweet Almond Oil, one pound and a half; two ounces of Alkanna root, (Radix Alkanna;) four ounces of white Wax; two ounces of Spermaceti, and twenty or thirty drops of Oil of Roses, which procure at a druggist's. Put the Alkanna root in the oil, and simmer over a slow fire for about three hours. In the meantime melt the white Wax and Spermaceti in another vessel. When the oil has got a very red color, take it off and strain it; then mix the other with it and when it begins to get cold stir in the Oil of Roses. Put it into a close vessel, that it may not loose its pleasant scent.

Wash the head clean with Castile Soap, and comb it well, that the skin may be as clean as possible; then rub the mixture about the size of a hulled chestnut upon the head, morning and night, every day.— If this is continued from three to nine months, it is sure to cover the head with a luxuriant growth of hair. It has never been known to fail, provided the person that used it was under fifty years of age.

A Remedy for Rheumatism and pains in the Joints.

Take half a pint of Spirits of Turpentine; half a gill of Sweet Oil; two teaspoonsful of pulverized Saltpetre, and two tablespoonsful of Tar; simmer all over a coal fire, till it commences to smoke freely.

Wash the painful parts with it morning and evening, using about two tablespoonsful at each time; but be careful not to get wet by rain. From three to ten drops may be taken inwardly during the external use of it, in the morning and evening.

For the Weed (so called) in the Breast.

Take one pint of Fish Oil, put into it as much Beeswax as will stiffen the oil to the consistency of a thick salve; melt the two articles together, add half an ounce of Venice Turpentine, and simmer a short time over a slow fire.

Spread a plaster of this upon a piece of linen or silk large enough to cover the breast, and renew it every night and morning. A small opening should be cut in the middle of the plaster, in order to let the nipple through and not prevent the child from sucking.

Another; which will Scatter the Hard Lumps in the Breasts of Nursing Women.

Take what is called No. 6, say two ounces, and strong Camphor Whiskey, one ounce; mix them well; warm the mixture into which dip a flannel rag, and lay it on the part of the breast affected, as hot as it can be borne; renew it whenever it gets cold and it will effect a speedy cure.

Invaluable Salve for Sore Nipples.

Take four ounces of Sweet Oil, half an ounce of

refined Borax pulverized very finely, two ounces of Spermaceti, half an ounce of white **Wax**; mix all together over a slow fire, stirring it often until the Borax dissolves; then let it get cold; if it should be too stiff, let it be melted again and a little more oil added; if not stiff enough, a little more Spermaceti should be added.

Anoint the nipples and the skin around them with the salve, morning, noon and night; always taking care to wipe the nipples clean before the child is put to the breast.

FOR THE WORMS IN CHILDREN.

There are several symptoms by which we are enabled to judge whether a child has worms or not, and in order to make it more discernible, I shall describe some of the symptoms.

The symptoms of worms generally are, a changeable color of face, sometimes very pale, sometimes red; a blueish looking ring under the eyes; itching of the nose, in consequence of which children often pick their nose or rub it; headache after eating; watering of the mouth at night; restlessness in sleep; gritting of the teeth during sleep; thirst in the morning; an inclination to fainting; giddiness of the head and a ringing noise in the ears; sometimes a craving appetite, at other times the sight of victuals can not be endured; bad smelling breath; sometimes sore gums, with vomiting; a feeling of oppression around the heart; pains in the stomach, particularly in the region of the navel; the stools, at times, are very loose and offensive, other times there is great costiveness of the bowels; the patient, notwithstanding a good appetite, remains lean and poor; is more restless and peevish in the dark of the moon or at the time of the new moon; grows fretful and sometimes delirious, with fits. Others get as stiff as a piece of wood; lay for a while senseless; wake up with a hard fit; grow delirious; go to sleep and upon waking or recovering, know nothing of what has happened. Some drink a good deal; others have a dry cough, resembling the hooping cough. Alexander Monroe says that the enlargement of the pupil of the eye was one of the surest signs of worms; another sure sign is, if when a person feels sick at the stomach, he gets suddenly better after drinking a glass of cold water. The surest sign of all, is of course, when there are worms thrown up, or passed off by the stools; and we must not expect to find all these signs in one person. It is sufficient when there are four or five of them present.— Enough has been said to enable a discerning mind to judge whether a child has worms or not. The remedy is:—

Take garlic, either the root or leaves, and the leaves of green rue, each equal parts; pound them together and press the juice from them. Of this give to a child six years old, fasting in the morning, two teaspoonsful, the same at noon and in the evening at bed time; continue this for about nine days, and upon the tenth day give a good dose of Salts or Castor Oil.— This course may have to be repeated three times; but it is a sure remedy for the worms, and will effectually destroy them if persevered in.

ANOTHER FOR THE SAME.

Take Carolina pink root, two ounces; Senna leaves, two ounces; Wormseed, one ounce; put the whole into half a gallon of water; boil it down to one quart;

then strain it and when settled pour off the clear liquor, which sweeten well. Of this give a child of four years old a tablespoonful every four hours, until it commences to operate on its bowels, after which it is to be given only twice or three times a day; always either one hour before or after eating, and continued until no more worms pass off. To children of older age the dose must be increased, and of younger years, diminished. This remedy I have never known to fail. If it should not operate upon the bowels sufficiently free, a little Castor Oil may be given occasionally.

SECRET REMEDY FOR THE TAPEWORM.

Take one fourth of an ounce of the powdered root of Male Fern; mix it with a glass of water and drink it, fasting in the morning, and repeat the same at bed time. Continue this for five days; then take the following pill the sixth day, fasting: Calomel, twelve grains; Resin of Scammony, five grains; Gum Gamboge, five grains; powder and mix the ingredients well and form them into a pill, by adding a drop or two of molasses and a little light bread. If this should not operate freely by night, it may be followed by a dose of Salts or Castor Oil. This dose is for an adult, and may be increased if the patient is of a robust habit, or diminished if of a weak constitution. The process may be repeated five or six times; during which the patient may eat freely of salt victuals, but drink as little as possible. This remedy has cured its thousands in Germany and France.

TO CURE THE RINGWORM.

Take linen or muslin rags and burn them on the steel part of an axe; when burnt you will, after blowing off the ashes, find a kind of greasy fluid upon the

steel; with it rub the part well. This should be repeated morning and evening, and continued for two
or three weeks, when it will surely produce a cure.
There are places in Germany where nothing else is
used for this complaint.

REMEDY FOR A DISEASE GENERALLY CALLED THE "SHINGLES AROUND THE WAIST."

Rub the parts affected with the Oil of Cedar, morning and night, for about two days. If this produces
a burning pain that can be no longer borne, the blood
of a black cat may be rubbed on twice a day, until
cured.

The rubbing on of cat's blood may seem ridicu-
lous in the eyes of some, but let them try it, and perhaps their ridicule will cease, when forced to admit
that there exist remedies in nature for the cure of diseases, the cause of which we are not able to explain.
Whether the blood of a white or brown cat will answer the same purpose or not, and why not, is not my
purpose to explain here; and any one anxious to
know may search the mystery himself. I have tried
the above; it has fully answered its purpose in giving
relief and performing a final cure, and what experience has taught me is good, I can conscientiously recommend to others; whether they laugh at it or not
is of little difference to me.

INDIAN CURE FOR A CANCER THAT HAS ROOTS.

Take one or two good sized white onions, pound
them well and make a poultice of them; lay it on the
cancer for twenty-four hours, after which take it off
and pull easy on the cancer, to see whether it is loose
or not; if it does not seem to be loose, let a fresh
onion poultice be applied for twenty-four hours, after

which try it again; if somewhat loose, then the root of the broad-leafed yellow dock, dried by the fire and finely powdered, should be sprinkled upon the roots of the cancer. Again renew the onion poultice, and so repeat every morning and night, pulling the cancer slightly every day, and sprinkling fresh powder on the roots until you can pull the cancer out by the roots. The pulling of it must be done carefully, so that the roots do not get torn. This remedy will sometimes take a cancer out in eight days; sometimes, if a large one, it will require from four to six weeks. When the cancer is removed, the wound may be healed up with any healing salve.

FOR SHORTNESS OF BREATH IN CHILDREN FROM 1 TO 10 YEARS OLD; SOMETIMES CALLED PHTHISIC.

Take two handsfull of the leaves of the plant called Motherworth, (the kind here meant has a square stem) fry it in about a tea-cupful of fresh, unsalted butter; then add to it two middle sized red onions, (red in the inside) sliced fine; frying it all together until the butter begins to look brown, taking care, however, not to scorch or burn it; then strain and let it get cold.

Bathe the child in warm water up to the arm-pits every evening; then wipe it dry and grease it well with the salve from the neck to the pit of the stomach, rubbing it downwards; repeat the same every evening before going to bed, continue it for four or six weeks, and a sure and safe cure will be performed.

FOR SHORTNESS OF BREATH IN ADULTS; CALLED ASTHMA.

Take half a pound of the green root of Swamp

Cabbage, (some call it Skunk Cabbage,) clean it well and slice it into one quart of Alcohol or French Brandy; add two ounces of Valerian root, (Radix Valeriana) let it stand for about two weeks in a warm place, shaking it occasionally; then strain it and let it settle, pour off the clear liquor and it will be fit for use. Of this a person above fifteen years may take one tea-spoonful morning, noon and night, mixed with a little water in which there has been a small quantity of assafœtida dissolved. The dry powder of the roots, half a teaspoonfull three times a day for an adult, is also a sure and safe remedy for the above complaint. The use of it has to be continued, sometimes, for three or six months. If about thirty drops of sweet Anis Oil were added to the Alcohol after it is strained, it would prove a valuable addition. The remedy is an oft tried one, and will only require perseverance to insure a favorable result.

REMEDY FOR PAIN IN THE BONES.

Take the inner bark of the prickly ash, say two good handsful, put it into one quart of French brandy, add one handful of the inner bark of quaking asp; let it stand for about two weeks in a warm place, shaking it occasionally. Take of the brandy, every morning and night, a table-spoonfull in wild cherry bark tea. Its use should be continued for two or three months, and the bowels kept loose during the time by occasional doses of Salts or Castor Oil. The above dose is for a grown person.

A SURE REMEDY FOR THE AGUE.

When the proper evacuations have been attended to, and there is no appearance of bile in the stomach, (which may be known by the formerly coated tongue beginning to look clean, the bitter taste in the mouth being gone, &c.,) take two ounces of Peruvian Bark, one ounce of Cream of Tartar, one ounce of Cloves, one ounce of Gentian Root; pulverize the two last, and mix all together and put them into one quart of French Brandy or good old Rye Whiskey; let it stand for three or four days in a warm place. Of this let a grown person take a tablespoonful every hour in tea of dog-wood bark, and continue the same three or four times a day for two weeks after the ague has disappeared. For children give smaller doses.

Any one with whom the spirits will not agree, may infuse the ingredients in half a gallon of water and simmer it over a coal fire for a few hours, then the dose for an adult will be half a teacupful every hour, and for a child from five to fourteen years old, one tablespoonful every hour. The infusion in brandy is, however, best.

This is a remedy with which the fever and ague has been successfully cured in this neighborhood, and in hundreds of cases it has never been known to fail.

A PREVENTATIVE FOR THE FEVER AND AGUE.

Take two ounces of Peruvian Bark, two ounces of Juniper Berries, one quarter of an ounce of Cayenne Pepper, one ounce of Rhubarb coarsely powdered, and infuse the whole into a half gallon of water; simmer it over a slow fire for about four hours, then add one pint of Rye Whiskey.

For adults two tablespoonsful, morning and night; for children, from two years old and upwards, from one to two teaspoonsfull will do, mornings and evenings.

___

To Insure Health and Prolong Life.

Take, for one week, two grains of white pepper, morning and night, swallowing them whole; during the week following, take four grains morning and night; the third week take eight grains morning and night, every day, and so continue, always taking three weeks for the course. A perseverance in this simple remedy will improve the health and strength gradually, give a good appetite and prolong life, if such can be accomplished at all. It is to be remembered that it is the ripe fruit of the pepper shrub, that is meant here, known generally to druggists as white pepper, and not the black pepper, sold in stores, which is the unripe fruit of the pepper shrub. Children may use half of the above dose.

___

A Certain and safe Cure for the Bowel Complaint.

Take a small dose of Salts or Castor Oil; when it has operated take one tablespoonful of the following tea every hour, until you have taken for six hours. Wait twelve hours, and if not relieved, repeat the process. Children from two years old and upwards, may take one teaspoonfull, increasing according to age, following through the same rule as above. No cold water should be given during the use of this remedy. The tea is prepared as follows:

Take one good handful of the bark of the root of black haw; boil it in one pint of sweet milk for about fifteen or twenty minutes, then strain it before using. This is a remedy never known to fail, though it may, in the eyes of some, appear simple.

For the Dyspepsia and Sick Head Ache.

After a good physic of Calomel and Salts or Castor
Oil, (or a good vomit may answer the same end) take
every morning, noon and night, of charcoal made of
green wood of the white walnut, as much as will lay
upon a small teaspoon, for nine days successively.—
After this time take another physic, and then repeat
the course of charcoal, and on the tenth day take a
physic, and continue in that manner from three to six
months. In the beginning it may give a little inconvenience, but after a week or two no inconvenience
will be felt whatever, and in the end the greatest benefit will be derived from it. The charcoal may be
mixed with honey, molasses, sweet milk, stewed ap-
ples, or something of the kind. It may be prepared
as follows :

Take the branches of the tree not exceeding two
inches in diameter; take off the bark and chip the
wood, which put into a close covered skillet or oven,
and heat the same to a red heat for about half an hour.
Then let it cool and powder the coal finely, leaving
it exposed to the atmosphere as short a time as possible. It may be kept in a close corked bottle. The
dose above mentioned is for an adult, but may be increased if necessary.

For Worm Fits.

Take of powdered Valerian root, one ounce; powdered Rhubarb, half an ounce; Magnesia, half an
ounce; mix them thoroughly. Dose for a child four
years old, half a teaspoonful three times a day, for about
two weeks in succession. For a child eight years
old, two teaspoonsful three times a day may be given
n tea or milk. If these doses should operate on the

bowels too severely, give them only twice a day; however they should produce a moderate effect upon the bowels, and if they do not do so, a little Castor Oil may be given every other day.

To Stop the Wound of an Extracted Tooth from Bleeding.

Sprinkle copper filings upon a portion of cotton large enough to fill the wound; insert it, and the bleeding will stop as if by magic. It is seldom that a repetition will be necessary.

For the Watery Eruption upon Children's Heads.

These eruptions often appear in the shape of small blisters, containing a sharp, watery, yellowish fluid, which burst open, spread over the head and form very painful and troublesomes sores, being of an itching and painful nature. This remedy will speedily remove them and prevent their return, if persevered in for some length of time after they have disappeared.

Give the child every three or four days, a dose of Salts or Castor Oil, and let it abstain from salt victuals and pork; in the meantime sprinkle finely powdered charcoal, made of green hickory wood, upon the place affected, renewing it every morning. Before this, however, the parts should be washed thoroughly with castile soap suds. The head of the child should be kept covered during the use of this remedy.

Splendid Eye-Water for Weak Eyes.

Take ten grains of Sugar of Lead and powder it very fine, then dissolve it in a half pint of rain water or creek water. In the morning and evening wash the eyes with about one teaspoonful of the mixture. Before using, the eyes should always be washed with cold, fresh water.

ANOTHER FOR WEAK, SORE, OR WATERY EYES.

Ten grains of Sulphate of Zinc, (white vitriol) dissolved in a half pint of rain or snow water, and apply as above. A Spanish fly blister laid on the back of the neck and effectually drawn, may also be of great benefit to watery eyes.

AN EXCELLENT COUGH SYRUP.

Take four handsful of Elecampane root, two handsful of Wild Cherry bark; boil in one gallon of vinegar until half boiled down; then strain and add three pounds of Loaf Sugar, and boil the whole to the consistency of a syrup. Keep it in well stopped bottles, and give, for a child two years old, one teaspoonful three times a day; for an adult, one or two tablespoonsful two or three times a day. This is an excellent remedy for coughs and colds of every description, applicable in almost all cases and at all times.

FOR DEAFNESS, PRODUCED BY THE WAX HAVING GROWN HARD IN THE EAR.

Wash the ear well with castile soap suds; then wipe dry and drop into it four or five drops of the grease of an eel; then insert in the ear, as far as possible, a wedge-shaped piece of Burgundy pitch, around which should be wrapped a little fine Bobinett, so that it may be readily withdrawn. Continue this, renewing it every morning and night for three weeks; then again clean the ear thoroughly, and repeat the same process, cleaning the ear every three weeks until a cure is performed. This remedy has cured deafness arising from the above cause, which had been of eight years standing in a man about sixty years old.

Opodeldock for Bruises and Sprains.

Take two ounces of clean white soap, slice it into one pound of Alcohol. Also: an ounce and a half of Camphor put into one pound of Alcohol. Let both stand for about six days, shaking each occasionally, after which pour the clear liquor from both preparations into a bottle or jar with a wide mouth, and add one drachm of the oil of Rosemary, stirring it well. Set it in a cool place, when it will soon become thick and be found an excellent remedy for sprains and bruises of all descriptions.

A Remedy for Mortification.

Take four ounces of Alum, four ounces of flour of Brimstone, one half pound of gun powder pulverised, mix all well together and sprinkle the affected parts with the mixture; or dissolve a tablespoonful of it in one teacupful of strong vinegar, and wash the parts with it three or four times a day. One-small teaspoonful of this mixture may also be taken inwardly daily as long as the outward application is continued.

For the Glanders in Horses.

Take Camphor, four ounces; Alum, four ounces; Saltpetre, four ounces; Rosin, four ounces; Crude Antimony, four ounces; Assafœtida, four ounces; Toemum Græcum, four ounces; Glauber Sals, four ounces; Flour of Brimstone, four ounces; Indigo, two ounces; pulverize it all together very finely, and sprinkle one tablespoonful of the mixture over the horses food three times a day. When the horse gets better give it only twice a day. Horses should be fed on wet wheat bran during the use of this remedy, and lime water given daily as a drink.

Salve for the Piles.

Take one drachm of Sugar of Lead, and twenty-five grains of Opium; reduce both ingredients to a very fine bowder, and mix it thoroughly with two ounces of fresh lard or butter; then anoint the parts well with it, morning and night; it will not only give great relief, but, if persevered in for a length of time, will perform a cure. Every six or eight days a dose of Salts or Castor Oil should be taken.

A Quick Remedy for Colic in Horses.

Take a portion of hair from the foretop, mane, and tail of the horse, burn it on some coals, letting the smoke go into the animal's nostrils. At first the horse will not like it; but in a few minutes will stand quietly to it. It will suddenly cure the worst colick, and is a remedy much practised in Germany.

A Healing Salve for Sores op all Kinds

Take one drachm of Sugar of Lead, finely powdered; White Wax, one ounce; Sweet Oil, four ounces; mix the Oil and the Wax together, stirring in the Sugar of Lead until cold. Spread a plaster and lay it on the sore, renewing it every morning and night; always washing the sore with Castile Soap suds before putting on the plaster.

Antibilious Pills.

Take Aloes, half an ounce; Calomel, one drachm; Gamboge, twenty grains; Ipecacuanha, twenty grains; Castile Soap, two drachms; Oil of Cloves, twenty drops; powder the Aloes and the Gamboge very fine; then add the Calomel and Ipecacuanha; after it is all thoroughly mixed add the soap, finely scraped; then drop the oil in and mix all well together, adding a lit_ tle water if necessary. Out of this mass form one hundred and twenty pills, three of which, taken at bed time, will serve as a physic for an adult; or for a very robust person, four of them may be taken. No cold water should be drank until after the pills operate two or three times.

For Suppression of the Menses.

If through cold the courses do not appear at the usual time, take two tablespoonsful of pitch pine knots, finely scraped; one handful of garden chamomile; put the two into one quart of old rye whiskey, and let it stand for nine days. Then, after a dose of Salts or Castor Oil, give one tablespoonful three times a day, every day, and bathe the feet in warm water every night. Continue this only until the menses make their appearance, when its use must instantly cease; for it is a powerful, sure and speedy remedy. Care must be taken not to use it in suspected pregnancy, as it will surely produce an abortion.

Suppression of the Menses in Child bed by Cold.

Make strong tea of green hemp leaves; give the patient half a teacupful every four hours, and in the mean time apply watm poultices, or wet warm rags to the abdomen. The tea must be discontinued as soon as the first signs of returning courses show themselves. The leaves may be dried and kept for winter use, when a few more should be taken than it green.

For Flooding, or too Great a Flow of the Menses.

Take two large tablespoonsful of the green buds of dog wood; bruise them, and boil about twenty minutes in one pint of strong vinegar. Then strain and give two tablespoonsful every half hour, until the flow moderates or

Another for Suppressed Menses, from Cold

Put two handsful of the bark of the root of Yellow Poplar, and an ounce of Aloes into one quart of French Brandy; let it stand for nine days, shaking it occasion- ally; then take one teaspoonful three times a day, every day, in a little Lovage tea, and bathe the feet in warm water every night. It must be discontinued as soon as the menses begin to appear again.

For the Itch.

Mix one drachm of red Precipitate with an ounce of hog's lard. With this annoint the elbow joints, groins and calves of the legs, morning and night. Take care not to get wet by rain or otherwise.

For a Burn by Water or Fire.

Take a good handful of unslacked lime; put it into a half gallon of water; let it slack and settle; then pour off the clear water and strain it. Then take about one pint of the water and mix with one pint of flaxseed oil, sha- king it well together; then annoint a linen rag well with the preparation and lay it on the burn, renewing it twice or three times a day. The patient should also, if the burn be large, take a dose of Salts or Castor Oil every three or four days, and avoid eating salt victuals. This will heal a burn rapidly and scarcely leave a scar.

Consumption and Spitting of Blood.

Take Gum Amoniac, one drachm; Sulphate of Cop- per, twelve grains; pulverise both very fine, and with a little molasses form the mixture into thirty-six pills, of these pills an adult may take one, morning and night; if costiveness of the bowels should come on, it must be re- moved by a dose of Salts or Castor Oil.

For the Bite of a Copper-Snake.

Take a handful of the leaves of the plant called Silver- weed, boil them about fifteen minutes in a pint of sweet-milk; then take the leaves out, lay them over the wound, and drink the milk. The application of the leaves boiled in milk, should be renewed every day.

Another cure may be had by mixing equal parts of Hartshorn and Sweet Oil, dipping a rag in it and laying it on the wound, renewing it two or three times a day.

A Sure, Safe and Quick Method to Break the Fever in almost any Disease.

Take a handful of Spice Wood, a similar quantity each of Dog Wood bark and Beech bark; boil together in half a gallon of water, until there is only one quart left; then strain and let the patient drink freely of it while it is warm. This will soon break the height of the fever and produce a moderate perspiration, upon which the drink prescribed must be immediately discontinued. The feet of the patient should be bathed in warm bran water, during the use of the drink. This is especially applicable in scarlet fever and measles, in both of which it will facilitate the eruption greatly.

For Rheumatism in the Limbs and Joints.

Take two tablespoonsful of the Jamestown weed, called by some, "Thorn Apple;" after bruising, fry them in a teacupful of fresh lard or butter, for about half an hour. Then strain, and anoint the painful parts with it morning and night. It may produce a sweat in some cases, but is sure to give effectual and permanent relief.

For Stiffness of the Joints.

Take an equal quantity of Fish-worm-oil and ground hog's fat; melt it together, after which add one half of rattlesnake oil and mix it well. Anoint the parts well with this, morning and night, for several days, and even weeks, if necessary.

Fishworm oil may be prepared by gathering the Fishworms, putting them in a bottle stopped well and sitting.

it in a warm place in the sun, or on a stove. They will turn to oil in four or six days, sometimes sooner.

For Difficulty in Passing Urine, in Small Children.

Bathe them to their arm-pits in warm water, and give flaxseed or parsely-root tea, or tea of water-melon seed, or of the rotten bark of the sour-gum tree. The bathing should be repeated every six or eight hours, until relief is found.

For the Bite of a Mad Dog.
A Remedy Recommended by Dr. Ingram, of London.

Immediately after the bite, to prevent the poison from incorporating itself with the blood, apply a hot iron, (not so large as to prevent its penetrating to the depth of the wound) to the part. The wound only needs to be burnt slightly, after which it should be rubbed with a little Sweet Oil and a salve or plaster applied to produce running, which will extract the poison.

In a period of six years, which the above named gentleman spent in the West Indies, he had a full opportunity of testing this remedy. The remedy deserves the attention of the public as well as physicians. as by it many valuable lives may be saved.

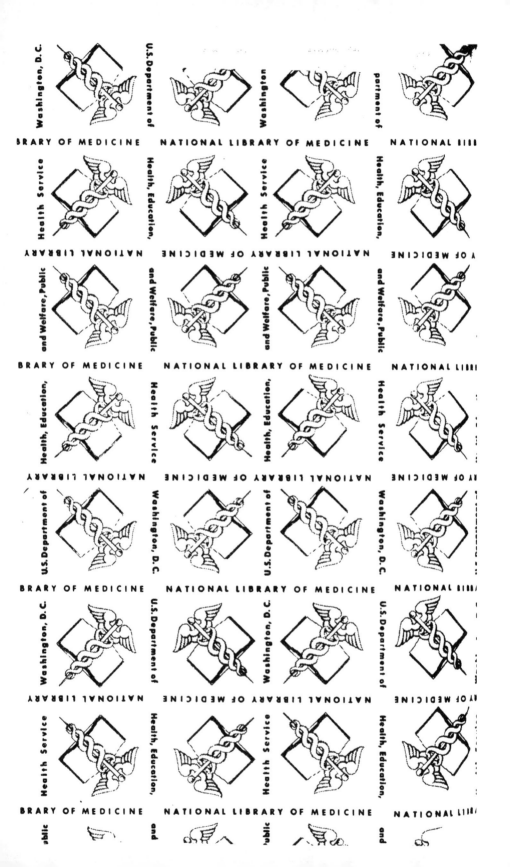

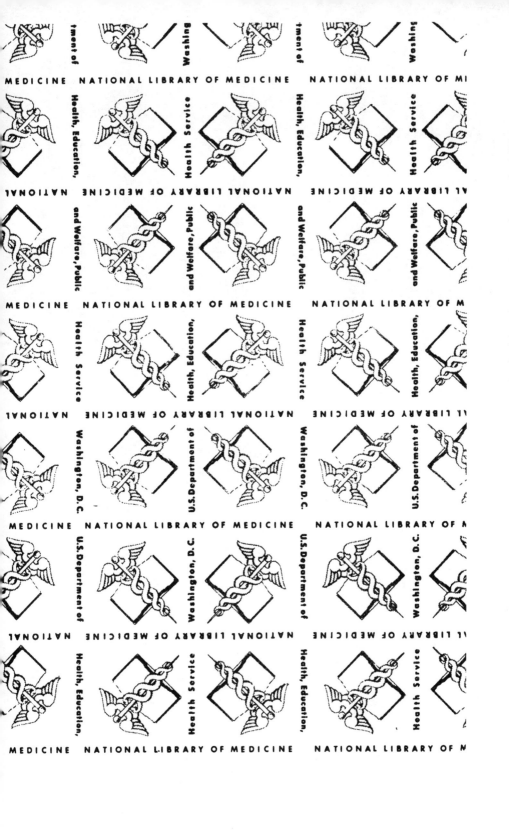